Praise for Mary Shouse and *Breaking the TIC Cycle*

CW01508956

"Mary's creative and sensory-driven approache
have helped my son tremendously. I recommend this book (and the
tools inside) to any parent of a child with tics, newly diagnosed or not."

Brenna D., mother of a 12-year-old boy with Tourette Syndrome

"Mary's ideas and approach combining self-regulation, awareness, and
new ways to manage tics has helped my son thrive. With her techniques, he was able to overcome vocal tics to meet his goal of attending
a symphony performance."

RoxAnne S., mother of a 9-year-old boy with Tourette Syndrome

"We were looking for the right support for our son with tics for years.
Once we discovered Mary and her holistic techniques for tic management described in this book, we saw his confidence skyrocket and his
anxiety decrease."

Silpa K., mother of a 12-year-old boy with Tourette Syndrome

"The tools and concepts in this book have helped me decrease my
tics to better live my life and have more confidence for the future. I
recommend Mary's compassionate and effective approached for people
with tics of any age."

Elias R., adult with Tourette Syndrome

"When our daughter was diagnosed with a chronic tic disorder, we
weren't sure what to do. With Mary's interventions, our daughter went
from having significant neck pain due to tics to being nearly pain free
in only six sessions with her techniques."

Brittany P., mother of an 8-year-old girl with a chronic tic

BREAKING THE

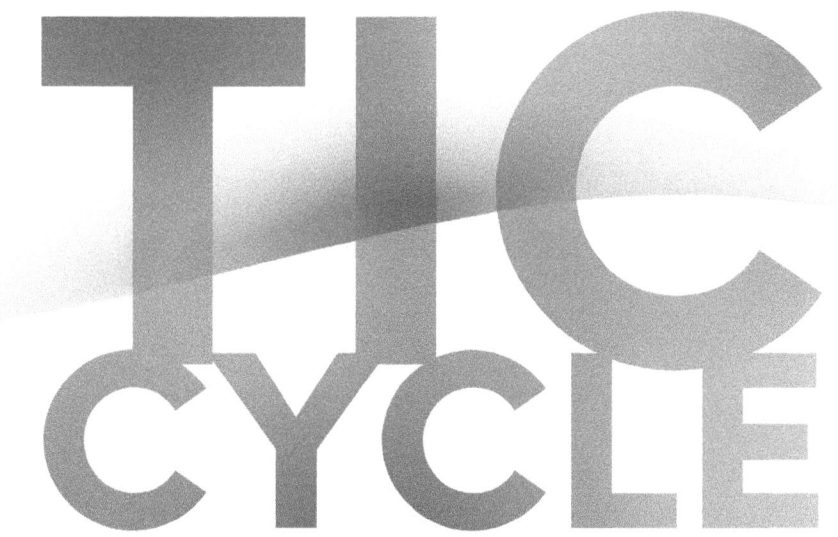

MARY SHOUSE, MS OTR/L

BREAKING
THE

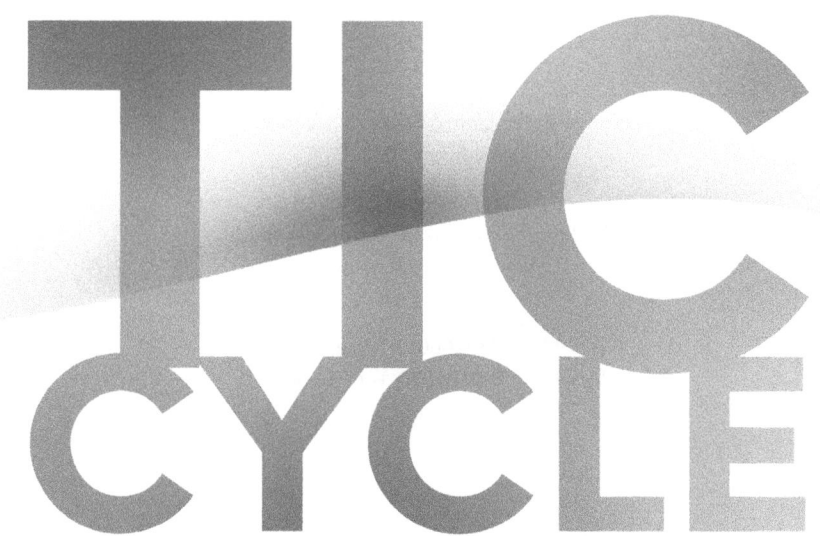

PRACTICAL SOLUTIONS

for Tourette Syndrome & Tic Disorders

Printed in the United States of America.
First edition 2023.

Cover and layout design by G Sharp Design, LLC.
www.gsharpmajor.com

ISBN 979-8-9894600-0-7 (paperback)
ISBN 979-8-9894600-1-4 (ebook)

To Jeremy, for always believing in me.
And to my wonderful clients, past, present, and future.
It is because of you that I will always do this work.

TABLE OF CONTENTS

INTRODUCTION

You can significantly reduce your tics by following ten simple and actionable steps. What?! How is that possible? In this book, I walk you through the exact steps I have used for years with my clients to help them manage their tics and live better lives. This book will give you actionable steps you can use today—without setting up expensive appointments with nutritionists or specialists with long waitlists.

As an occupational therapist and provider of behavioral therapy for tics, I have worked with clients with tic disorders of all ages, helping them achieve tic management to be able to learn, work, and thrive. I fell into this specialty on accident when employed at a pediatric therapy clinic. I had two new clients who both had diagnoses of autism and Tourette Syndrome in the same week! What are the chances of that? It was then that I realized that I needed more information to really help these clients and eventually pursued training in Comprehensive Behavioral Interventions for Tics through the Tourette Association of America. Since then, I've been able to combine my knowledge of the sensory system, the mind-body connection, and incorporating the power of internal motivation and functional problem solving to obtain amazing results for my clients.

Whether you have had tics for the last fifteen years or have been recently diagnosed with Tourette Syndrome, you know that having tics can be debilitating, embarrassing, painful, and inconvenient. They stop you from being your authentic self in social, school, and work situations. You may worry that tics will prevent you from being able to get the job you want (or keep it).

If you are a parent of a child with tics or Tourette Syndrome, do you lie awake at night wondering what the next day, week, or years will bring? Are you anxious about what will happen to your child at school—about whether or not they will get bullied or excluded because of their tics? Even more upsetting, is your child asking you if there is anything you can do about their tics, and you feel totally helpless about what to do next?

If you are reading this book, you've likely already tried medications and Googled all the natural remedies and diets you can find, but the tics persist. Maybe you were told by your primary care doctor or neurologist to just "wait and see." Maybe you were given a prescription, but the tics are getting in the way of all areas of your life, and they don't seem to be getting any better.

In this book, I have organized and structured all of the most effective strategies, tools, and techniques I use into a step-by-step process that anyone can follow to manage their tics. In fact, using the techniques I outline in this book, I have had some clients reduce their tics so significantly that they are hardly noticeable. I will guide you through the process with simple steps that will work whether you are a child, adult, or teenager and no matter how long you've been experiencing tics. Even if you fall into the category of having more than one neurodiversity, such as being autistic or having ADHD, these tools will work for you.

Combining components of research-backed traditional therapies (such as Comprehensive Behavioral Interventions for Tics) with other tools that connect body and mind for self-regulation, you will achieve more progress in managing your tics than ever before. What's more, once you find the techniques presented that help you, you can go back to them time and time again if new tics pop up. Your uncertainty and anxiety about the future will be reduced as you realize that you have a trusted game plan that you can use anywhere and anytime.

In this book, I will guide you through my tested process for effective tic management that really works. With step-by-step guidance, practical tips, and problem-solving tools, you'll learn:

→ how to use sensory inputs and insights to reduce tic triggers
→ what to do (and not to do) during a "tic attack"
→ how to determine if your child needs an Individualized Education Plan or 504 plan at school (and how to get one)
→ what to do if tics are affecting you at work (and what your rights are)
→ whether or not behavioral therapies are right for you and how to find a therapist
→ the top six myths people believe about tics
→ how to improve your autonomic nervous system regulation to increase your inner resilience to stress and anxiety
→ how to bring up tics with family, friends, and colleagues

If you have been looking for effective tools to manage or even eliminate your tics, this book is for you. No matter how long your tics have been around, this book can help you gain mastery over your tics and clarity about your next steps.

1

THE MYTHS PEOPLE BELIEVE ABOUT TICS

Before I was an occupational therapist specializing in tic disorders, all I knew about tics were that they were involuntary movements and sounds. The only treatments I had heard of were medications. In both my graduate and undergraduate courses, I learned a ton about autism, developmental disabilities, and other conditions. What I didn't learn about was how to help people with tic disorders and Tourette Syndrome. As of May 2023, Centers for Disease Control statistics report that about one in fifty children has a persistent tic disorder (including Tourette Syndrome), and they also indicate that this number is likely too low, as diagnosis for tic disorders are often delayed or not made at all due to lack of awareness.[1]

Are you as surprised as I am that an estimated one in fifty children have a tic disorder? Where are all the walks, the fundraisers for research, the specialized therapy clinics, the family and community meetings, the training and books for parents and clinicians? I soon realized that, although the Tourette Association of America has many resources for families and providers, their reach was not enough. Not every state has a Center of Excellence, and I've met many clients and their families who reported that they felt like they were grasping at straws for care and struggling to find clinicians and therapists with expertise in tic disorders.

Once I learned about this discrepancy in care and knowledge in providers, I decided to increase my involvement and support. It wasn't fair to these people that they had to take this journey all alone, not knowing that there are millions of others all around them who also have tics.

And there are so many myths and stereotypes. When I talk to a new or prospective client, they always ask me a million questions, which I love to answer. Many of them have to do with myths that they believe or have heard about tics.

In our society, much of the general public's information about tic disorders (and OCD as well) is literally a punchline and *totally wrong*. Most people associate Tourette Syndrome with outbursts of swearing, or coprolalia, but in actuality, less than 10 percent of people with Tourette Syndrome have this type of tic.

As we know that we are up against an abundance of unhelpful and just plain wrong information, what can we do and where do we go to get accurate information about them. And what about help to manage them?

American, Canadian, and European guidelines all recommend Comprehensive Behavioral Intervention for Tics (or CBIT, an effective behavioral therapy we will discuss later), as first-line treatment for children and adolescents with tics.[2] However, an overwhelming majority of primary care doctors and even neurologists are unaware that this therapy exists, let alone recommend it to clients. And even when they do, finding a therapist is extremely tough (and yes, I'll give some recommendations about how to find a therapist later).

In order for the world to change, and for therapy, tools, and support to be accessible to all, we first need to address these myths. What are they?

MYTH #1: There is nothing you can do for tics besides medication.

Because many doctors begin and end the discussion of tics with recommendations for medication, people believe that it is the only way to manage tics. Why are more physicians not recommending therapies or other alternative treatments for tics and Tourette Syndrome? Unfortunately, as I reported earlier, most therapy education programs, whether you are an occupational therapist, physical therapist, social worker, or psychologist, are not preparing providers to help people with tics. This makes it much more difficult to find medical and health professionals that are skilled in treating people with tic disorders and for doctors to refer out to them.

And since the medical establishment in the United States is closely connected to the pharmaceutical industry, most of the research and trials for treatment for tic disorders are based on profit-producing medications and drugs. They are able to be covered by insurance, easy to prescribe, and can be made widely available.

This needs to change. Although medications for tics and Tourette can be absolutely life-changing for some, many people struggle to benefit from these pharmaceuticals. And yet, we have evidence-based interventions that are not being recommended to them. I am here to help sound the call, to get more providers interested in this type of work, and to help people with tic disorders themselves become advocates to support others. The time has come!.

MYTH #2: Tics are involuntary, so therapy won't work.

Although tics are involuntary movements, twitches, and sounds, you may have noticed that they can be very suggestible. Emotions, environments, and routines can have a great impact on the severity and frequency of tics, which can be confusing. What does this mean? It means that we can use this information to our advantage when helping a person manage their tics.

The same attributes that can be frustrating about tics (that they are so variable and occur in different environments) can help a therapist and client carefully craft a tic management plan with a good ability to predict when certain tics may happen. And because these factors can be reasonably consistent, once identified, they will help a person prepare for when and where new tics may surface. Part of therapy for tics also involves addressing nervous system arousal and emotional regulation, which can dramatically impact a person's tics as well.

MYTH #3: My tics are too severe for anything to help.

No matter how severe your tics are, there are many interventions that you can try that will help. This doesn't necessarily mean that your tics will completely go away but that the options, interventions, and therapies available can play a huge role in improving your quality of life.

One of the major wins that I have with clients is helping them overcome barriers (whether they are emotional, physical, or logistical) to the life they want to lead. Once a person achieves some progress on their journey, it is amazing how their mindset shifts to see new possibilities in life.

After years of feeling hopeless, using my techniques, they begin to participate more in life to an extent that they didn't believe they could. Some of my clients even use their newly acquired skills to help others, transforming their personal journeys into advocacy for the greater good. That begins a new cycle of positivity that continues to grow and affects other areas of their lives, such as in relationships and opening up new work and school opportunities.

Increasing autonomy (a person's personal concept of independence and abilities) can help someone with even the most severe tics gain momentum and start a positive cascade of activity that provides purpose and meaning.

MYTH #4: My tics have been going on for twenty years. It's too late to do anything about them.

One of the most common concerns I hear from new clients is worries that their tics have been going on so long that there is no hope for them. They have resigned themselves to the way things currently are and have determined that, unless a new miracle medication comes down the pipeline, there are no options.

Have you heard of the concept of neuroplasticity? Neuroplasticity allows our brains to form and reorganize synaptic connections, especially in response to new learning and new experiences. This is the same phenomenon that allows us to learn how to speak a new language at fifty or go from falling off a surfboard to becoming a big wave surfer and loving it. Because all of our brains have this new capacity for change, transformation, and acquisition of new skills, there is no age limit to when you can improve your tics.

Even if you have had tics your entire life and have tried every therapy, medication, and natural remedy on the market, it does not mean that you won't benefit from the techniques and tools I'll share. Although there hasn't been evidence to affirm brain changes after therapy related to tic disorders, there is plenty of evidence to support actual changes in brain connectivity for other conditions (PTSD, etc.) after therapy. Why not harness this power of our brain's ability to change right now?

I want to reassure you, no matter how you feel right now and no matter how long it's been, there is hope for you. Even if you never end up working with me directly, it is my deep desire that the new knowledge you will get from this book will propel you on your journey to improvement and will steer you toward the quality of life you deserve.

MYTH #5: I've heard of CBIT therapy. Isn't that just suppressing tics?

It is a fact that some tics are suppressible, or able to be "pushed down" or "held in," at least for a short amount of time. This may lead people to think that, in therapy, a client is learning to suppress tics. One of the core components of Comprehensive Behavioral Interventions for Tics, Habit Reversal Training, is actually helping people do the opposite. It is helping them create new habits and automatic actions that teach the brain to get used to, or habituate, the feelings they have before a tic.

One of the first things I teach my clients in therapy is the inconvenience of suppressing tics. Children often understand this, as in most classrooms teachers are prompting students to "keep eyes on me," "keep hands and feet still," and "voices off." What is someone to do with a motor or vocal tic to avoid getting in trouble or lectured? Kids learn very quickly that suppressing tics is a good way to keep them from looking "weird" or being called out by the teacher. So what's the downside? If you think of a tic as energy that needs to get out or be expressed, what do you see as a parent when your child gets off the bus or in the car after school? A tic explosion, that's what! Then this pattern gets reinforced day after day, month after month, and instead of learning new skills that are helpful and reduce tic intensity and frequency, they get very good at suppressing and releasing tics, causing more stress.

It is imperative that, when going through therapy and the activities presented there, you understand the difference between suppression and learning. You will realize that your brain is actually making new connections and pathways during therapy. It is learning new tools, new ways of being, and new ways to handle your most common triggers, *not* just suppressing tics.

MYTH #6: I have autism/ADHD/OCD, so therapy for tics won't work for me.

A common hallmark of having a condition such as Tourette Syndrome is having what is called "The Tourette Triad.[3] This essentially means that not only do you have Tourette Syndrome but you also have co-occurring conditions, typically ADHD and OCD. It is thought that these three developmental disorders relate to a common brain network or area called the basal ganglia. This area of the brain has to do with inhibition, and these conditions are all related to challenges with inefficient inhibition. These problems with inhibition of movement or sounds (as in motor or vocal tics), inhibition of perseverative or intrusive thoughts (as in OCD), or difficulties with impulsive behaviors (as in ADHD) are all related. So what does that mean? It means that, in order for therapy to be effective, it needs to address these relationships and teach ways of managing these challenges that are simple and practical.

When you add in the likelihood of having an additional neurodiversity, such as autism, the challenges in treating tic disorders can be daunting. People with autism often have differences in sensory processing as well as differences in bodily awareness and self-management in social situations. It is essential to look at these differences through a new lens, not one of problematic deficits but one of strengths and acknowledgement of unique neurologic makeup.

A good program for tic disorders will help a client understand their uniqueness and how it can be helpful to them, rather than a barrier. It will emphasize the benefits of having a different brain and will look for solutions that allow the person to be who they are, not to "mask" their differences so that they can fit in with the people around them and society.

Who are the best professionals to do this? Occupational therapists! As an occupational therapist, I have had extensive training in the nuances and physiology of the sensory system and how it influences a person's behavior and self-regulation. To overlook this crucial part of our physiology leaves behind essential factors that impact tic management.

If you are worried about your therapy not being neurodiversity-affirming, remember that your perspective on your conditions and challenges is what should be driving your therapy and interventions. You will see in the suggested interventions in this book that I take an approach to help you highlight what you are already successful in and want you to be able to advocate for your unique way of being and individual priorities in all of your care.

How do we address these factors in the interventions presented here and ensure that we are neurodiversity-affirming?

→   Ensure that therapeutic interventions and coaching are focused on the client and their wants and desires, no matter their age.
→   Look to expand upon a person's innate talents, preferences, and ways of being.

→ Address sensory differences and needs and respect differences that serve the person functionally, *including stimming*!

→ Eliminate masking or suppressing differences in communication, coping, and sensory needs to promote fitting in or not looking "weird."

→ Address the person from a holistic perspective, meaning acknowledging body, mind, community, as well as present and future needs and goals.

→ Modify techniques and ways of communicating strategies for better comprehension (such as using more concrete visuals, video modeling, etc.).

By now, I hope I have addressed some of your concerns about why these interventions (and therapy) might not work for you. You've seen how, despite having multiple and sometimes complex diagnoses, there are still very effective ways to reduce your tics and massively improve your life. Now is the part you've been waiting for. How do we get there? Keep reading. I am excited to help you officially start this journey.

2

THE PRINCIPLES OF SUCCESSFUL MANAGEMENT

I f you are reading this book, you are likely looking for ways to help with your tics now! You may be unable to find a therapist who can help you, you could have too many things going on in your life to commit to therapy, or it is not in your budget at this time (I understand completely). My clients all differ in terms of readiness for change, the co-occurring conditions they have (and the severity), their background history with tics, and why they are seeking treatment. I address all of these in their specific plan of care, or as I like to call it, the Tic Success Plan! Despite the fact that every person I see is very different, there are seven basic principles that guide my therapy with each client that will be essential for you to know.

Principle 1: Determine if CBIT Therapy Is Right for You

As a CBIT therapist, I'd love nothing more than to help everyone who walks through my door using CBIT therapy. One of the things that brings me indescribable joy in life is seeing a person who has been struggling with tics long term improve dramatically in six to eight weeks. I seriously live for this! However, despite this, not everyone is ready for CBIT therapy to manage their tics. And this is important for you to know, whether you are a parent of a child with tics or a prospective client yourself. Why is not everyone ready? What's the big deal?

First of all, CBIT is a behavioral therapy. This is different from a medication-based therapy. In a behavioral therapy, it is essential that the person participates as fully as possible in order to be successful. What does that mean? It means this:

→ A child who is unaware of their tics is not ready for CBIT. You can't improve something you are unaware of, whether it is due to reduced body awareness or challenges in outer focus.

→ A teen who refuses to participate or has to be "forced" to come to CBIT therapy is not ready.

→ A person whose tics do not bother them is not ready, and they wouldn't need treatment either.

→ A person who does not want to do therapy, for whatever reason, is not ready and should not participate in CBIT. And, as humans with autonomy, no one should require us to participate in any kind of therapy that we don't want to, whether you are an adult or a child.

Who else is not ready for CBIT therapy:

→ Someone who is undergoing a significant, stressful transition, such as a new job, new school, divorce or separation, or moving to a new place.

→ Someone who has severe co-occurring conditions that may be more impactful than the tics, such as severe OCD symptoms, anxiety, depression, suicidal ideation, or severe ADHD. Although people with these conditions can benefit from CBIT, it is crucial to make sure that the timing is right and that other symptoms are not going to make participating in CBIT therapy harder than it needs to be. I always remind parents that preservation of self-esteem in a child or teen is imperative, and undergoing a therapy that they are not ready for would be unsuccessful. Even worse, a child or teen could blame themselves for not succeeding in therapy. That is the last thing any parent or therapist wants for a child.

→ An unstable family situation where both parents are not on the same page about therapy or tics and will not support the child in the way they need. Family support is an essential component of a child's success, and it just won't work if parents will not or cannot help the child.

So now that we know who is not ready, who *is* ready and is a good candidate for CBIT?

These are the type of people who I see and who are ready for CBIT therapy:

→ They want to participate in therapy and may have been asking, "Mom, is there anything else we can do for my tics? They are really bugging me."

→ They have enough awareness, physically and mentally, of their tics and how they are impacting their life. This could be as simple as, "My eye blinking tic keeps making it hard to remember where I was on the page when reading my book."

→ They are managing co-existing conditions reasonably well. We know that many, many people have tic disorders and other conditions at the same time (more on that later). But if anxiety or depression is debilitating, that should be addressed first to get optimal benefit from CBIT.

→ They have a stable family situation, and both parents are on the same page about therapy and will support the child. Family support is an essential component of a child's success, and parents play a very important role of coach in therapy.

→ They are able to commit to at least six weeks initially and then several intermittent sessions in the future.

Principle 2: You Can Address Co-Occurring Conditions as a "Backdoor" Approach

So what if you or your child falls in the category of "I have a significant co-occurring condition that is not being well managed"? I have some good news for you! If you are struggling with tics and have severe or significant anxiety, depression, OCD, or ADHD, this could be a key to reducing your tics without undergoing CBIT therapy!

I call it the "backdoor" approach to reducing tics. Often, people struggle more with the symptoms of their anxiety or OCD than they actually do with tics. One of the things that I hear all the time from parents is when a child has a new, more understanding teacher, or they finally resolve some of their OCD symptoms through treatment such as ERP or counseling for anxiety, their tics decrease significantly.

Consider this: What happens to your child's tics when they are out of school for the summer? No long homework assignments, no sitting still at a desk all day, no stress from the combination of sports, piano, and learning their least favorite subject. Do their tics improve? For some, they improve to the point where the parent is no longer interested in having their child pursue CBIT therapy!

As an adult, what happened when a short-term stressful event was resolved? Think about a time such as when you finally got in the groove at a new job, your mother-in-law left after a long visit, you patched things up with someone you had a disagreement with. Did it improve your mood and your outlook on life, with a sense of more hope for the future? Likely, your tics decreased as well and you felt they were less intrusive.

Addressing co-morbidities through targeted and individual therapy that can change your mental state and patterns can make a big difference in how your tics present and how much they bother you. Does this mean that this reduction of tics will last? Maybe. Depends on some of the situations and scenarios we will address in the next few sections. But don't discount the role that other conditions play in the frequency and severity of your tics—managing them could be an absolute game changer.

Principle 3: Stress at Work or School Makes Management Harder

This is an obvious statement, and you are thinking, "Duh! Of course dealing with stress at work or school makes my tics worse! What do I do about it?" When I meet with an adult or parent for the first time, one of the first things we discuss is how work or school is going. When a person has significant tics, they will often report, "Not well."

In a school setting, there are often several common factors that are contributing to the exacerbation of tics in the environment, including being bullied or excluded from peer groups, being made fun of due to tics, or struggling academically and not receiving adequate or appropriate help. When you are going through therapy to manage tics, these challenges can make things much harder, and that is why they should be addressed.

Each of these situations has a unique way to address them, but I will first tell you about a particular strategy that has *really* been helpful for many of my clients as well as youth in my community who are being excluded or bullied: having a Youth Ambassador from your local chapter of the Tourette Association present to your child's class or school.

In addition to being a CBIT therapist, I am also the Youth Ambassador Coordinator for my state's chapter of the Tourette Association of America. (I told you helping people with tics was my life's calling; I do it for fun as well!) When requested (and if available) you can have a Youth Ambassador (a teen who has tics or Tourette Syndrome or is an ally) come do an eye-opening and engaging presentation about what it is like to have tics. The students go through a simulation to see what it is like to have tics, and boy, do they enjoy it! And they love to talk about it. Next, they get to ask the Youth Ambassador all about what it is like to have tics. They get to hear firsthand what it is like to have tics or Tourette and how they can support people around them. At the end of the presentation, the Youth Ambassador leads everyone in a pledge to commit to be supportive and caring to the people who may have tics or Tourette

Syndrome. The child in the classroom with tics doesn't have to be involved or acknowledged in any way if they don't want to.

The first time I witnessed the power of this small action was when I accompanied a thirteen-year-old Youth Ambassador to the classroom of a fourth grader. His classmates were very receptive to the presentation, and the magical thing was, this experience not only helped the student who was struggling, but it helped the Youth Ambassador as well! He became more confident in sharing about his tics and how he wanted to be responded to, authentically. I don't hesitate to say that this endeavor was equally helpful for both.

After the presentation, the student's mom emailed me to say that he was having a completely different experience at school (a much more positive one). His classmates were more supportive and ignored his tics, as the "elephant in the room" had been addressed. Now this is not to say that every child wants a Youth Ambassador to come to their school for a talk, or that this is the solution to bullying. However, if one small event like this can provide a ripple of understanding that grows, it may be something you should consider. Of course, I highly recommend it! How do you even find a Youth Ambassador program in your area? You can find one by searching on the TAA website: www. tourette.org.

What about the struggles of academics and how that impacts tics? We will talk more specifically about how to access academic, emotional regulation and organization support at school further in this book. But for now, you must know that even if tics don't appear to be impacting a child or teen at school from the outside, there is still a good chance that they are.

One of the reasons has to do with the concept we spoke about, called "tic suppression." Many of the teachers I have spoken with either in the classroom or at IEP meetings will commonly say, "I've never seen Johnny tic at school. His tics are not impacting him here at all." Can I say, as politely as possible, "Wrong!" Unfortunately, this is a common misconception among educators and people in general. If they can't outwardly see someone struggling, especially with tics, then they must not be having them or they must not be a problem. But as a parent or adult with tics, you probably know many kids get through the day without issue by suppressing, or holding in, their tics as long as they can. How well would you be able to learn and retain new information if you were trying to suppress something *all day long?* It would be a herculean task!

They hear continually from teachers' statements like, "Eyes on me," or "Bodies are still," or "Voices off," and need to comply in order to prove that they are "listening." Don't get me started on the need to move in general due to sensory needs and ADHD. When a child is suppressing tics at school to make sure he doesn't get held in from recess (yes, I have recently worked in the schools, and even now when we understand how important movement is to focus, that *still* happens!) it is *very* hard to learn new concepts while controlling their bodies and can make tics worse. I'll provide some recommendations later about how to address these school issues (and more).

Similarly to school, work is a place we go daily, and for most of us, a minimum of eight hours a day. When you are having a difficult time with the emotional stressors of work, such as dealing with an overwhelming workload, or having to deal with bullying from coworkers (and yes, adults can be bullies too), this can make managing tics and succeeding in therapy very difficult. I've got some practical tips and advice that will help in the Tic Management Roadmap.

Principle 4: CBIT Alone Is Often Not Enough

If you've read this far, you know how passionate I am about making sure that anyone who may benefit from CBIT has access to it. But unfortunately, it is far from a panacea. Have I had clients who did not gain much benefit from CBIT? Yes, and all CBIT therapists will tell you they have too. That is one of the reasons your therapist will (and should) thoroughly make sure you are a good candidate before beginning. You don't want to waste time, money, or end up disappointed. Many of my clients complete CBIT therapy while taking medication for tics or ADHD or emotional regulation as well, and this is absolutely fine and very common. So when I say that CBIT alone may not be enough, this is what I mean.

Life in these modern times can be overwhelming, to say the least! We are dealing with so many stressors that seem to increase exponentially each year, such as a barrage of information from all sources (information overload), greater need to be "connected" via social media (and the resulting fallout from comparing and feeling more isolated than ever), inflation that means the same bags of groceries cost more than ever, the new worry that AI will take over all of our jobs... Need I go on?

And these are just some of the concerns adults face that are on the top of my mind. Teens and kids have other stressors, as you know, and there is no pause button. And this is all on top of having a tic disorder. Because of this, you may need more than just a series of CBIT sessions to help you manage your tics, as the extra stress does a number on our nervous systems and thought patterns. Don't worry, I'll make sure to help with some recommendations on this later as well.

Many of my clients benefit from having a counselor that they see regularly. Even if you don't need to see them weekly, and choose to have monthly check-in sessions, that can often be very helpful. Some of the issues that can be associated with tic triggers are ones that need attention from a mental health therapist. Learning new, effective coping strategies with effective mental frameworks for dealing with concerns can be a critical part of tic management.

I often recommend to my clients that they have an established "support team" that is connected to the person or their child. There is nothing worse than trying to find a counselor or talk therapist in the middle of a crisis. The same can be said for trying to find a new psychiatrist; they are in short supply and waiting lists can be long.

If you have a co-occurring condition along with your tic disorder—and as we've identified, many people do—one piece of your tic management puzzle is making sure that you have access to the right therapies for your needs. Don't wait on this! You won't need to see a therapist all the time if you don't need to, but having one "on standby" will go a long way for your piece of mind and overall tic management.

Another piece of your overall tic management plan is having regular stress-relieving practices (yeah, you figured that was coming). They don't need to be hard, a big deal, or even another thing on the endless to-do list that feels like work. That won't last and you won't be able to keep it up long term. (Remember that time you committed to yoga four times per week? Talking to myself here!) Let's keep it so simple you can't not do it! I will provide easy-to-do, sensory-based practices in the Tic Management Roadmap.

Principle 5: Addressing Sensory Needs Is Essential, Even If You Think You Don't Have Any Sensory Needs

The first time I ever saw the iceberg image from the Tourette Association of America, I had been assigned to evaluate an autistic child with Tourette Syndrome for occupational therapy at the clinic where I worked. I immediately started Googling when I got home, and the first resource I discovered was the website for the Tourette Association of America. When I downloaded the iceberg PDF my jaw dropped!

Here's a description of the image: A large iceberg floats in the water, with the header "Tourette Syndrome: Tics are just the tip of the iceberg". Above the waterline, you see the following: motor tics and vocal tics. This represents what the average person sees and understands about Tourette Syndrome. Under the waterline, you see the following: learning disabilities, behavioral issues, disinhibition, sleep issues, depression, ADHD, handwriting difficulties, obsessive compulsive behaviors, social communication deficits, anxiety, impulsivity, sensory processing issues, transition issues, and executive functioning deficits.

When I saw these labels, I knew that I had so much to offer people with Tourette Syndrome. I started brainstorming and thought about all of the ways that I could help this child that would possibly soon be in my care. Many of these concerns and issues are within the expertise of occupational therapy, especially when it comes to helping with sleep issues, sensory processing differences, and handwriting difficulties.

I've been working with clients with Tourette Syndrome for years, and in that time I have seen the ways that sensory processing differences and challenges can impact tics in people of all ages. Even if you think that differences in sensory processing do not affect you, if you have tics, think again.

What is sensory input anyway? The term "sensory" has become quite a bit of a buzzword recently. Many people don't fully understand how our complex sensory systems are helping to gate, filter, and manage all the inputs around us. We now know that in all brain states, even in unconscious ones, sensory processing of internal and external inputs is happening in our brains. It is like the breathing of oxygen and the beating of our hearts, forever occurring 24/7, 365, silently in the background.

For those with average and efficient processing, much of the sensory information coming in is typically pushed out of our conscious awareness, and for good reason. Scientists have proposed that our sensory systems are picking up information flow at a rate of eleven million bits per second, however, they report that we can only perceive around forty bits of information per second.[4] So not only do our brains (in collaboration with our sensory system) help us perceive information about the world inside and around us, but they also help us filter and make sense of salient information. They also allow us to disregard information that is irrelevant, which is just as crucial.

If you know someone who is autistic, or are autistic yourself, you may already understand that sensory issues can be highly correlated with specific diagnoses (like autism). But you may not have realized that sensory processing differences also disproportionately impact people with tic disorders. If you have functional tics or Functional Neurological Disorder, it is well established in the literature that sensory experiences can both trigger and exacerbate tics and negative symptoms. There have been similar findings in Tourette Syndrome.[5][6] This may come as no surprise to you, and you may have observed how sensory inputs impact your own tics or those of your child. I have had clients tell me that they tic more when they are hot or in the sun or that they are more sensitive to sounds, smells, and other people being in their close proximity.[7] [8]

All of this evidence indicates that, when working on a tic management plan, it is important to screen for and address sensory-based impacts. In my work as an occupational therapist, I have had the most success for children and adults with helping them to identify their own sensory differences and sensory-based tic triggers, while guiding and supporting them to find modifications and compensatory strategies that reduce or eliminate them. You may be surprised to learn how common sensory inputs impact your tics once we put a spotlight on this area.

In the Tic Management Roadmap, I will introduce screening tools as well as a sample tracking and intervention form to help you create these strategies on your own. Even if you don't have a tic disorder and are reading this book to support someone else, it will be helpful for you to undergo this exploration for yourself.

Principle 6: Setting Up a "Tic-Neutral Environment" Is Essential

You may have heard your child's neurologist recommend ignoring his or her tics. Why is this? This principle goes hand-in-hand with the next principle, which is not accidentally reinforcing tics. How does creating a "tic-neutral environment" reduce the likelihood that you will reinforce tics? Why is it a best practice in the home and school environment (and work for that matter)? And what exactly does it mean?

A tic-neutral environment is as simple as it sounds: essentially you are not remarking about, commenting on, or actively trying to soothe away a person's tics. The person is allowed to tic as they need to, as much as they need to, without your interference or calming. This is easier said than done in a family environment with a lot of people. You know that tics are involuntary movements and sounds. But you've also learned that they are highly influenced by people, activities, emotions, and sensory inputs. Because of this, rather than asking a person directly to try to tic quieter, to stop ticcing, or to go in another room to tic, it is much more helpful and advisable to simply ignore the tics and let them happen as they need to. As we will see, even doing something helpful for the person (such as encouraging them to relax or take a break from hard work due to ticcing) can reinforce the tic. In fact, research demonstrates that tic-related talk can actually increase tics.[9] Douglas Woods, one of the leading experts in Tourette Syndrome, recommends the following to establish a tic-neutral environment:

- → Do not react to your child's tics.
- → Do not express frustration with your child's tics when he/ she is present.
- → Do not lower your expectations for your child due to tics.
- → Do not be the "tic police."

The one exception to this rule is when you are undergoing CBIT therapy and are actively working on managing a specific tic. In that case, you are helping the person as a coach, encouraging them in their exercises and reminding them of the exercises they have. In all other cases, ignoring the tics is the right way to go. While ensuring a neutral environment at home, there are things you can do proactively or during an upswing in tics:

→ Provide or encourage a positive distraction without mentioning tics, such as changing the environment. "Hey, why don't you go in the backyard and toss the ball around for the dog? She looks bored!"

→ Remind the child or teen of active, engaging activities they can do around the house rather than passive activities (watching TV or being online or on their phone). "Remember I got you that Diamond Art Kit? Why don't you make a new picture?"

→ Help your child with physical movement, particularly if they don't like sports and need encouragement in this area. "Can you walk down to the mailbox and get the mail?" or "I saw a new game you can play while you are jumping on the trampoline. You can toss the ball against the wall and catch it while you are jumping. Wanna try it?" Or even take a five-minute movement break: "Taylor Swift dance party time!"

Along with the creation of a tic-neutral environment, it is essential that you do not inadvertently reinforce tics. Huh? Why would I want to do that? Well, obviously you wouldn't. Unfortunately though, I have seen it many times in my practice by well-meaning parents. Here are some of the ways you can inadvertently reinforce tics.

You can reinforce tics by allowing your child to "escape" from a non-preferred task or activity due to tics. Here is an example I have seen in some of my own clients: Shawn sits down, begrudgingly, for his daily piano practice. As soon as he sits on the bench, his motor tics flare up, seemingly out of nowhere. Instantly, he is twitching, rocking, and now is unable to keep his hands on the keys, let alone play. His mother compassionately sees this and tells him he doesn't have to practice today, that he can try again tomorrow. And wouldn't you know it, right before piano practice the next day, it starts happening again! Without realizing it, Shawn's mother has inadvertently reinforced his tics. But wait, if tics are involuntary, how is that possible? I'll let you in on a not-so-secret secret that we've previously discussed: tics are influenced by our environment, emotions, and nervous system arousal state. Even though Shawn can't help that he has tics, his emotional state (the strong negative response to practicing piano) is collaborating with his brain to trigger the tics. Once all the stars are aligned (setting, time of day, people around, arousal state) the tics start to increase. So how can we circumvent this?

Here's how: Even if Shawn's tics are coming in fast and furious, it is not a reason to not hold him accountable just as you would anyone else. You can be sensitive to the fact that they are really bothering him, and he is just as frustrated as you are about this. However, sending the message to his brain that tics are not a "hall pass" to avoiding the things that are most challenging will help to eventually curb his brain's connection between all those aligned "stars" and the tic frequency.

How can we do this? If you notice that Shawn is ticcing before or during a nonpreferred or difficult task, you can remind him that sometimes that may happen when he has to do something hard, and that's okay. He can set a brief timer while staying in the area (still sitting on the piano bench) to calm and distract himself and potentially use a coping skill he has practiced and is familiar with. After the designated time (usually five to ten minutes) he will continue the activity as best as he can, even if the tics flare. Keep repeating this cycle until the tic flares during those emotionally charged activities lessen (and they will). This strategy can be used in other similar circumstances, such as during homework time. You can even explain the strategy to your child to help prepare them if they are experiencing this. Here's what I coach my families to say to their children:

> **Parent:** "Yesterday we noticed that your tics started to get pretty bad during homework and they were really frustrating you. Remember that? Today, we are going to try a new strategy to help teach our brain that it is stronger than **(Insert Task)** so that you can keep doing the things that are important.
>
> If you notice that your tics are really bugging you and making it very difficult for you to keep working on your homework, let's give your brain a little break. You can stay here at the table, and we can try the box breathing your therapist taught you (or progressive muscle relaxation, putting a weighted pad on lap, etc.). We will set the timer for five minutes, and after that you will keep going, even if it gets tough. Your brain is very smart and looks for patterns, so it will learn this new strategy quickly. Let's teach it the pattern of grit!"

If you've never read Angela Duckworth's book, *Grit*, or seen her TED talk, I highly recommend it! It has nothing to do with tics, but the concept of teaching and embracing perseverance, or being "gritty" is very beneficial. It may even become a common word in your family's vocabulary. This term articulates the concept of continuing on when things get tough and not quitting. I often model this language with my two sons and deliberately identify times I show grit, or am gritty. Boy, do we have to do that a lot as adults! Like when I keep trying to learn how to parallel park. I don't have one of those fancy cars that can do it for me. But I'll get it, and I am teaching my boys that even adults have to persist in things that are tough, unpleasant, and uncomfortable. Please know that I am in no way minimizing the distress and pain that can be caused by tics, but this concept is a vital one to learn, tics or not. It can be very helpful.

Another way to not inadvertently reinforce tics is to change an aspect of a routine where tics are continually triggered. If you or your child is experiencing an increase in tics at the same time, in the same place, with the same demands, with the same people, try to alter one or more of the conditions or sensory inputs. You can try to practice piano in a different place (move the keyboard to a different room), try to complete it at a new time, or try to complete it standing rather than sitting. Try listening to some quiet background music, or light a candle with a smell you like. I encourage you to experiment with these and see if they help!

Principle 7: Nervous System Regulation Is a Small Hinge That Swings Big Doors

Most people have heard some basic information about our nervous system. It's pretty widely known that we have two divisions of our autonomic nervous system: parasympathetic and sympathetic. They are often correlated with our "fight or flight" response (sympathetic), and the "tend and befriend" or "rest and digest" responses (parasympathetic).

What you might not know is that in people with tic disorders, there are often autonomic nervous system differences. In my own work with clients, the most common differences I have seen are increased heart rate, nervousness, and anxiety.[10] The good news here is that we can help regulate the nervous system using low-level modalities (as simple as breathing) as well as the evidence-based ones that I offer in my practice, such as biofeedback.[11] [12] More on biofeedback later.

Why do we need to harness the power of our nervous system to reduce and manage tics? The simple answer is that using effective interventions that alter our nervous system function can operate as a remote control for tics. Imagine that: using a remote control to reduce your tics! Well, in actuality it isn't quite as easy as pushing a button. However, these interventions and modalities are still extremely helpful and should have a place in your tic management plan. The great thing is, you can alter your nervous system activation using simple, free tools you already have access to, or you can choose to try more sophisticated interventions. The choice is yours, but either way, the evidence is there—learn some and use them! I will help you decide what type of interventions might be best for you (or your child) in the Tic Management Roadmap. And remember, many of these interventions can be done remotely if you are interested in having me be your guide.

3

THE HOW-TO:
FOLLOW YOUR OWN TIC
MANAGEMENT ROADMAP

"I am so tired and exhausted dealing with these tics! We keep trying and adding new meds, titrating doses, and still nothing. I guess we'll just have to deal with these tics forever (or cross my fingers my child is one of the ones that grows out of them)."

I cannot even tell you how many times I have met with a parent and they sat next to me and cried. (And if I'm honest, I've even cried with them at times. Those parents who have worked with me know. I'm a sensitive empath and Enneagram Type 2; I can't help it.)

When your life is revolving around managing tics and the fallout, and it seems like most people don't understand, it can be isolating, hopeless, and discouraging. For some people, just getting a diagnosis takes a long time.

So now that you've got the diagnosis of Tourette Syndrtome or a tic disorder, what do you do? Here is the part of the book you've been waiting for. Or maybe you skipped to this part as soon as you opened the book. (I do that too!)

The following sections will identify each step to creating your own tic management plan and are important components of your own journey to success. I have outlined them in the order in which I would typically recommend them to my clients. You will have work to do, but if you follow these steps, I can assure you that you will make significant progress in reducing your (or your child's) tics. Are you ready? Let's go!

Ten-Step Roadmap for Tic Management

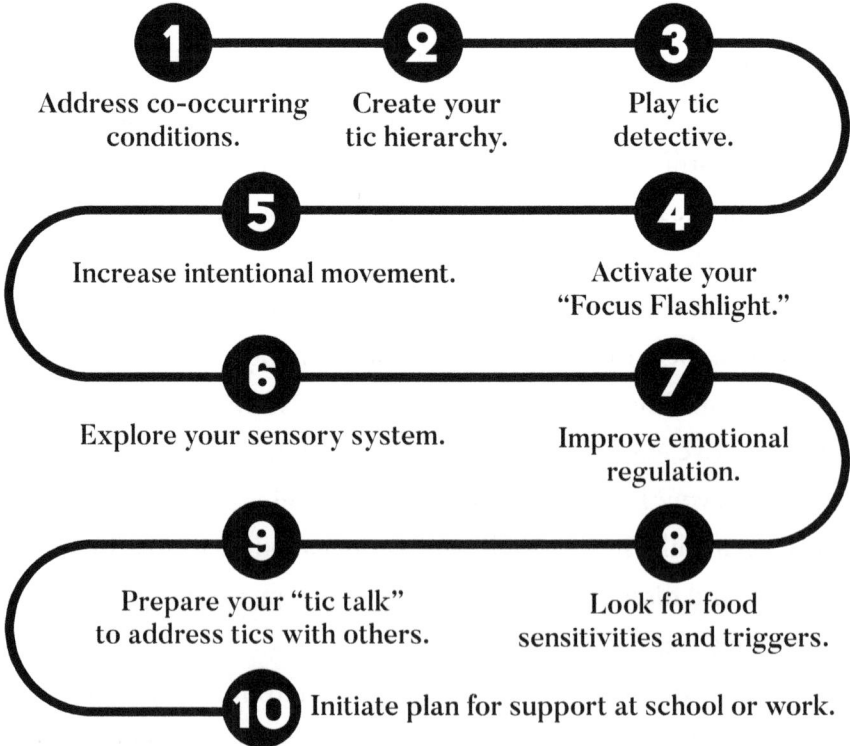

1. Address co-occurring conditions.
2. Create your tic hierarchy.
3. Play tic detective.
4. Activate your "Focus Flashlight."
5. Increase intentional movement.
6. Explore your sensory system.
7. Improve emotional regulation.
8. Look for food sensitivities and triggers.
9. Prepare your "tic talk" to address tics with others.
10. Initiate plan for support at school or work.

Step 1: Address Co-Occurring Conditions.

How many people have a diagnosis of Tourette Syndrome along with another condition, such as ADHD, OCD, or anxiety? A lot! In fact, you would be in the minority if you only have a tic diagnosis. So why am I mentioning this as the first step in our Roadmap to Tic Management? Because understanding whether you have a co-occurring condition and whether that should be managed first is a crucial step, and I don't want you to waste any time or energy.

So let's get to it. Answer the following questions using the scale provided.

	Not At All	Somewhat	A Lot
If you or your child has ADHD, do you have difficulty with task completion, to the point where you are frustrated or overwhelmed at least a few times per week?			
If you or your child has ADHD, do you struggle with impulse control that interferes frequently with your relationships (including family, friends, or authorities such as a boss or teacher)?			
If you or your child has ADHD, do you struggle with getting through the school or workday on a regular basis?			

Do you experience frequent
recurring, intrusive thoughts,
images, or urges that cause
distress and anxiety?

Do you feel compelled to
perform certain repetitive
behaviors or mental acts to
alleviate anxiety or prevent
a feared event from occurring?

Do you spend excessive
amounts of time engaging
in rituals or mental
activities, such as counting,
checking, or organizing?

Do these thoughts and behaviors
significantly interfere with
your daily life, relationships,
or occupational functioning?

Do you or your child frequently
experience excessive worry or
apprehension about various
aspects of your life, such as
work, relationships, or health?

Do these worries significantly
interfere with your daily
life, relationships, or
occupational functioning?

If you answered "A Lot" to several of the statements and questions, you may have another condition that is impacting your mental health (and indirectly, your tics). I do recommend that you seek guidance to find out if making progress on these symptoms would be helpful.

This is the first step to managing tics, as attention, regulation, and mood can impact them significantly and make it difficult to benefit from other interventions and therapies.

Remember, this quiz serves as a guide to help you plan your next steps and does not replace a professional diagnosis. It's important to seek guidance from a healthcare provider or mental health professional for a comprehensive evaluation and personalized recommendations based on your specific situation.

Step 2: Create Your Tic Hierarchy.

After we've established that your next step should be working through the activities in this book, you will start the creation of your tic hierarchy. What is a tic hierarchy? It is simply a list of the most current tics that are impacting you or your child and how bothersome they are. This helps you to target and drill down to the tics that are going to move the needle the most.

Here is how you complete the hierarchy.

Tic Hierarchy Instructions

Think about the last two weeks. Write down the tics that you have noticed (or noticed in your child). Use the chart to assign a number to the tic from 0-10 to rate how much this tic bothers you and write it down. You can use the downloadable chart at my website, www.helpfortics.com, to help you assign the number if needed.

Tic or Tic Symptom You Have Had in the Last Two Weeks	How Much Does It Bother You? (0-10 Rating Scale)

Here is a list that I find helpful if you are having a hard time remembering your tics. You can go through the list to jog your memory.

Using this list of body parts for motor tics, do you have any tics that affect the following areas?:

Motor Tic Body Parts List

Do you have any tics with your eyes?:
- → Eye blinking
- → Eye movements
- → Eye rolling
- → Eyebrow movements

Do you have any tics with your nose?:
- → Nose movements
- → Nose scrunching
- → Nostril flaring

Do you have any tics with your mouth?:
- → Mouth opening
- → Mouth stretching
- → Lip smacking
- → Teeth grinding or biting

Do you have any tics with your face, head, or neck?:
- → Facial grimace or squeezing
- → Neck movements
- → Head jerk/movements

Do you have any tics with your arms, shoulders, or hands?:
- → Shoulder shrugs
- → Arms shooting out
- → Finger or wrist movements

Do you have any tics with your abdominal muscles, legs, or feet?:
- → Abdominal tensing
- → Leg, foot, or toe movements

Vocal or Phonic Tic List

Do you have any vocal tics, such as sounds (animal sounds included), words, or phrases you repeat, or parts of words?

Do you have any tics that relate to breathing in or out, coughing, sniffing, or snorting?

This list is definitely not an exhaustive list of tics, but it will serve to help jog your memory to write down the tics that are most annoying, embarrassing, or painful. Once you've created this list, you can move on to Step 3 with the most annoying tic in mind.

Step 3: Play Tic Detective.

Part of the interventions I use in therapy for tics is a component called a Functional Assessment. What's great about this component and why it is included is that it helps to identify factors inside and outside of us as well as their consequences that may be influencing and encouraging tics. You can complete this assessment on your own to discover your own hidden patterns and reinforcers. Trust me, it will be extremely helpful for you. Let me tell you a true story of one of my clients that emphasizes just how important this step is.

I had recently begun working with a teenage girl named Lucy who was a sophomore in high school. We started by determining what her tic-related hassles were and why she wanted to go through therapy to reduce her tics. She identified that having tics at school was very upsetting for her. I probed the situation further, asking specific questions about which classes she seemed to tic more frequently, which classmates were in the class, where she sat, whether she liked the teacher and subject, etc. She was able to narrow things down and reported that in math class she had often had a loud vocal tic that would make people turn around and stare. She said she liked math a lot, and her teacher was very nice and helpful. She noted that she had friends in the class, and the homework load was not too bad.

So far, not a lot of information was pointing to anything specifically helpful. When I asked her where her seat was and who sat around her, her eyes widened. She almost looked like she was in a cartoon when a character has an idea and a lightbulb appears over their head. She said she sat in the front row, which she liked, and had even requested to sit there at the beginning of the school year. However, she said that her school had lost a geometry teacher suddenly, and her school's idea to make up for the lost instructor was to videotape her teacher giving the lecture. This video was then streamed to students in another classroom. As she sat in the front row, she was often in view of the camera for everyone to see. She reported that, since the recorded lectures, math was much harder as she spent a great deal of time in class suppressing her tics, especially the vocal tics.

Yes! We finally had a nugget that might be able to help! I spent some time explaining to her how this might be influencing her tics, and she responded that she thought for sure it was but hadn't considered it before. I let her come up with some ideas that may help to modify this situation and listened. She said that she wanted to ask her teacher if she could move to a new seat that would still be somewhat near the front but out of view of the camera. We role-played how she would ask her teacher, what she wanted to say, and how she wanted to say it. Her homework for the following week was to have the discussion with her teacher (at an opportune time) and report back any differences she noticed with the tics in math class.

The next week when I saw Lucy, she was triumphant! She eagerly told me that tics in math class (more specifically the vocal tics) went from a 9 out of 10 severity scale to a 2 out of 10, just by changing her seat! She said that her teacher was receptive to the change, and she had discussed the situation as we had practiced. Now keep in mind that when we decided to modify things in math class, we framed the changes as conducting an experiment. We determined together that moving her seat may have an impact and measured subjectively her experience before the change. This modification was viewed with neutrality, as it was just another part of looking for puzzle pieces disguised as dominoes to knock down—dominoes that may be able to have a larger cumulative impact. Another benefit of this specific scenario was that it gave Lucy a genuine opportunity to advocate for herself on her own terms.

How can you try this on your own or with your child? It is important to remember that your mileage may vary as far as the impact of what you modify or change, but it is a step that should absolutely not be skipped no matter what!

Here are the step-by-step instructions to performing your own Functional Assessment, or as I like to call it, Playing Tic Detective.

Step 1: To make this process easier, download your free Tic Detective Worksheet from my website, at www.helpfortics.com. Complete your tic hierarchy as directed. Choose the target tic (only one) that is most impactful at this time. This process is always performed on a single tic basis. Make sure it is a tic that is noticeable to your child and that he or she dislikes; otherwise they will not have any intrinsic motivation to complete this activity, and it will be very difficult.

Step 2: Determine or review the current level of distress related to this tic using the 0-10 scale already mentioned.

Step 3: Write out on the Tic Detective worksheet you've downloaded why this tic was chosen and why it causes upset or distress. Be as specific as you can. Does this vocal tic make it hard to go to a place where people are supposed to refrain from talking or making sounds (like a movie theater)? Do people look at you or comment when this tic happens? What do they say? Although asking these questions can be difficult, the more specific you are the easier it will be to track changes and remember your "why."

Step 4: Here is the part where you try to find the antecedent (the things that happen before this tic occurs). You are going to be looking for clues in the Tic Detective Investigation and then looking at hidden expectations (or rules, unwritten or overtly expected) and factors in the environment (such as people that are present or not present), just like a real detective. You want to gain as much information as possible, and no detail is too small! It is at this time that I like to get out a real magnifying glass for my pediatric clients to really get them in the spirit of detective work!

Step 5: You will use the worksheet provided to first find some antecedents (things that happen before the tic) related to situations or settings. Go down the list and checkmark the situations or places that this particular tic is bothering you most or is most frequent or intense in relation to other places or settings.

Step 6: Next, write down what the tic is like during this situation or setting. Give examples of what it looks like and how it bothers you while you are in the situation or setting. Remember, this gives us a clear picture of how it is impacting here and provides more motivation for change.

Step 7: Go down the list, gathering clues and labeling the following:

  a. Who is present? Think family members, teachers, friends, classmates. Is there anyone pertinent that could be a partial clue (your BFF, your arch enemy, or the most annoying boy in your class, etc.)?

b. What are the rules or expectations in this setting or situation? How do you feel about them? Note any strong feelings or emotions. (I hate going to PE; we always have to do sit-ups in front of everyone and it is so embarrassing!)

Step 8: What happens after the tics in this situation or setting? (If it happens during PE, do you then sit out the game on the benches? Do you keep going with the sit-ups?) Write this down.

Step 9: Look over your Tic Detective Worksheet. What stands out to you, as a parent or adult with Tourette Syndrome? Include your child in this process. What do they notice? Write down your observations in this format:

Tic Detective Investigation Results

I have noticed that when I am in/at **(identify place/setting/activity)**, my **(specific tic)** gets worse or is more bothersome. When this happens I usually **(write down the next action or consequence, such as, I get to take a break, I leave the room, I don't have to go to the grocery store, etc.).**

My sneaky brain likes to make connecting patterns all the time, even when I am not aware. In order to stop my sneaky brain's connections, when my tics get worse at/during **(place/setting/activity)**, instead of **(write down usual course of action)**, I will do the following: **(write down a new, different consequence)**. This will help my brain break the link between what usually happens that accidentally makes my tics worse.

Step 10: Implement the new consequences with as much consistency as possible. This is a time when I may offer an external reinforcer during this change. I think of it like rewarding myself with fancy new headphones once I have been able to follow my running routine for a few weeks to keep myself going. Even though my real reward is my increased cardiovascular fitness, the external reward helps keep me motivated during this new routine/change. You or your child may need a reinforcer too.

Here is an example of a completed Tic Investigation Result Worksheet that a child completed with a parent:

> I have noticed that my fist slamming motor tic gets worse when I sit at the table for dinner. When this happens, I usually take my plate and eat in the living room on the edge of the couch because it's a softer surface than the table. Sometimes I surf on my phone. In order to stop my brain's sneaky connection between sitting down to the table and increasing my motor tic, instead of going to the living room to eat, I will try the following changes:
>
> 1. Creating a pre-dinner calm-down routine. My mom will let me know fifteen minutes before dinner is ready, and that will be my cue to listen to my favorite song on my headphones and get my squishball from the drawer and relax.
>
> 2. When I sit down for dinner, I will sit at a different place at the table. This will help "trick" my brain, as it changes the usual pattern.
>
> 3. I will set a towel or foam mat down under my plate.

That way, when I have my slamming tic, it will be much quieter. This will also help "trick" my brain because the noise the slamming makes will be different.

4. I will eat at the table. Even if I tic while sitting there, I can put my fork down, talk with my family, and then pick it up again when I can. It might take longer to eat, but that's okay.

What you will often notice using this approach is that because the antecedents and consequences are noticeably different, your brain (or your child's) responds with less tics in that situation. It will be uncomfortable at first, as all changes are, but feeling some discomfort is a sign that your brain is changing—and the tic cycle is being altered. Even if it feels weird, keep going until you see some signs that your brain is no longer linking the antecedent to the consequence.

Step 4: Activate Your "Focus Flashlight."

"I never tic when I am swimming. Or when I'm playing basketball." my eleven-year-old client said to me. "Why?"

"Great question!" I said. "You have already figured out two special ways to use your mind to manage your tics. One is called your "Focus Flashlight," and the other is called "The Movement Controller." They both work kind of like the video game controller on your PlayStation, directing your brain to focus on what you want it to. Do you want to learn more about them and how powerful they are?"

"Yes!"

You may have also observed this phenomenon. When you (or your child) are engaged in something that you enjoy, particularly a physical activity requiring movement, the tics often lessen. Let's explore more about why this happens and how to harness this tool to help you manage tics.

If you have spent time on Google, you may have read that people with Tourette Syndrome and OCD have differences in a circuit of the brain (with a very long name!) called the cortico-striato-thalamo-cortical circuit. This circuit controls movement execution, habit formation, and rewards.[13] However, newer research demonstrates that more widespread parts of the brain are affected as well, including parts of the brain that are activated when we are thinking about our inner world and not the external environment and networks that help us decide which things around us are worth our brain paying attention to.[14] [15] Even the cerebellum plays a role in the sensation of tic release (or premonitory urges).[16]

Although it is helpful and interesting to know this information, what can we practically do with it? The first tool that is meaningful for my clients to understand (and simple for kids and adults) is the concept of the flashlight of attention, or as I call it, your "Focus Flashlight."

Essentially what this means is that we all have an inner flashlight that allows us to pay attention to various things outside of our body in our environment and also the sensations and feelings inside of our bodies. If you have ever experienced doing anything in a "flow state" then you understand the power of the Focus Flashlight. You may have felt rapt attention and went without eating or drinking, without focusing on anything but what you were doing. The sensation of time stood still. I personally know people who can get in this state while coding, rock climbing, writing, painting, or sculpting (and even playing Dungeons & Dragons). During times of flow, although you may not have intentionally turned on your Focus Flashlight, it was on and shining bright on the things outside your body that had your full attention. These are times when you may have noticed that your tics were completely silent, almost like they were turned off with a switch. How convenient! On the other hand, you may have noticed that when your Focus Flashlight was turned on and shining inward (say you are bored and sitting in a quiet waiting room with nothing to capture your attention), your tics may have increased significantly. How inconvenient!

So we can see clearly that, by turning on a flow state or by shifting attention outwardly rather than inwardly, we can use this as a tool to manage tics. Writer and researcher Steven Kotler, author of several books on flow and founder of the Flow Research Collective, believes that we can activate flow in some of these ways:

1. **Introduce novelty.** What is novelty? Something new and unusual that seems interesting to the brain and captures attention. One way I introduce novelty for my clients is to use Lego bricks to build things without direction, using their own creativity and imagination. Examples include the following prompts: "Can you make a tic-tac-toe board that we can play with out of the Lego blocks? Think about what your house looks like. Can you make a Lego model so I can see?" As adults we can introduce novelty by trying a new activity (one that won't be too hard to master). My husband has enjoyed the just-right challenge of using Woobles crochet kits for beginners. (Google them; they are adorable!)

2. **Cue curiosity.** One of the easiest and simplest ways to provoke curiosity in kids is to go outside and explore the world around them, at a tiny level. Look down, get on the ground. What do you see? Are there any bugs you didn't notice before? In this field of clovers, are all of them the same, or are any different? Science kits and experiments can also foster curiosity, even if they are as basic as using food color in water with an ice cube tray to mix and make new colors. How often does your child get to do that? It can be messy but fun! And for adults, think about some of the things you already do; can you do them differently. Do you have a curiosity list? This can be great for planned distraction and even getting yourself in flow. Is there a question that pops into your mind while in the shower, laying down at night, or driving? Add it to a curiosity list, and research it or explore it when you need distraction.

3. **Triggering dopamine through mastery.** Think about how good it feels when you are playing sudoku and you get an

answer right, and then you get three correct! That's the kind of feeling of mastery we are talking about. How about that rush when you are crocheting your cute little penguin, and you finally get the beak right and he's looking like more than a blob? Simple mastery through a just-right challenge (not too hard, not too easy) will keep your flashlight focused outwardly and heading toward the flow state.

Once you can predictably see the connection between using your flashlight of attention and how it changes your tic intensity and frequency, you have a tool that you can use at will.

Do we need to always keep our flashlight focused outwardly? No. Introspection, noticing our inner feelings, and attending to our inner world is a vital part of being human. Inner focusing can also be a tool for managing tics, as we will discover in Step 6: Explore Your Sensory System.

But once you've found the ways that your attention influences tics, when you are having an episode of significant tics, ask yourself, "Where is my Focus Flashlight now? Can I shift it?" and see for yourself the benefits.

Step 5: Introduce Intentional Movement.

How about the connection to movement? Does physical movement play a role in tic management?

There are several studies that demonstrate that increased physical activity correlates with a reduction in tic intensity and improvement in quality of life. In one study, researchers compared children with Tourette Syndrome and examined those who took an average of twelve thousand steps per day versus those who took less.[17] Those who walked at least twelve thousand steps per day reported lower vocal tic intensity, as well as rated aspects of their quality of life as greater than the group who did not have as many steps. Other studies report even simple movement, like sweeping floors or playing table tennis, had an impact on tic intensity as well.[18] And, as you probably already know, exercise can provide significant reductions in anxiety symptoms too.[19]

As a human species, our overall incorporation of movement seems to reduce each year as more and more technology exists that reduces our need to move (think robot vacuums, etc.). So even if you don't have tics, chances are you could benefit from more movement and likely don't get the recommended daily amount. Although more research needs to be done to examine the link between tic reduction and physical activity, there are many benefits that we can reap today, so let's do it!

What are some easy ways that you can add exercise and movement to your daily routines for tic management? Here are a few:

1. Instead of sitting down while you are talking on the phone, walk around or fidget with something. Same with kids; while they are playing Roblox on the

computer or watching TV, encourage them to stand. (Did you know that there are cheap hacks online to transform any desk into a standing desk using a simple Ikea side table?)

2. Place a rocking footboard under your desk or band on your chair legs. This works great for children too. Not only are your feet getting massaged, but it allows for movement of your lower body while you are getting things done.

3. Have your kids bring in the groceries. The heavy work of carrying in bags serves to provide proprioceptive input to the joints and ligaments while being a meaningful activity.

4. Brush your dog. You would be surprised how much pleasure this gives you (and the dog!). It has a double-dose benefit of promoting movement as well as bonding with an animal that is becoming calmer by the minute, influencing your nervous system as well. (My preference is to relax with my long-haired guinea pig Molly.)

5. Build in walking breaks into your day if you work at a desk and sit a lot. Can you get up and move every two hours at least to refill your water and take a few laps around the kitchen or office? All the steps add up. Same for your child at school. Are they permitted to walk around as needed? Are movement breaks built into the day, and how frequent are they?

6. Replace your chair with a yoga ball. I like the kind with a back support (also prevents falling off). Gentle

bouncing is not only helpful movement but has a calming effect on the brain. Think about the type of soft bouncing we do when we hold a baby. For kids I often recommend things like a wobble cushion on the chair so that they can shift weight as needed for calming movement while seated. A quick Google search will show you that there are tons of options for seating that promotes movement. Pick one and try it out!

7. Take a Swiffer break. I know, I know. Not exactly fun (well, maybe if you are a kid). But this has two benefits; you get the movement from walking around to Swiffer the floor and the satisfaction of seeking all the dirt and crumbs you've picked up. It's a win-win!

8. Wear a step-tracking watch. You would be surprised at how motivating it is to know how many steps you take each day. This can be a good idea to promote awareness to your movement, unless you think you may start to become too fixated on your step count. You can use it to set your timer for movement breaks and then try to take a few hundred steps before you sit down again (go get the mail, take that pile of clothes to donate to the trunk of your car). For kids, they can also use a step counter and use their "step break" to see how many steps they get carrying their belongings back to their room, putting their laundry away, or walking the dog around the block.

9. Encourage fidgeting. Rather than trying to stifle small movements in an attempt to "pay attention," use the

power of small movements to manage attention and allow energy movement. Here are some unobtrusive ways to fidget that will help your body and mind:

→ Stand while working. Whether you are an adult at work or a child at school, standing requires you to make small, continuous weight shifts that are controlled bodily movement.

→ Doodle on paper while working or listening

→ Tap foot on floor, tool or pencil on tabletop, or fingers on a surface

→ Chew gum, especially while sitting

Power of Rhythmic or Repetitive Movement

It is no secret how the use of repetitive movements can calm the body. That is why we rock babies side to side in a predictable way or subtly rock back and forth while standing and waiting. Our vestibular system (the sensory system that helps us with balance and body position) becomes activated and helps to calm us with linear, repetitive movement.

We can use the power of rhythmic movement to regulate our nervous system and, in doing so, help to calm tics. Many of these examples are simple, and you may wonder how effective they are. Introducing controlled repetitive movements on a consistent basis is counter to what we actually experience day to day. We no longer chop wood or carry items back and forth long distances, but our bodies and nervous systems still crave those types of movement.

Here are examples of rhythmic and repetitive movements that you can add into your day to provide proactive calming to your nervous system:

→ **Swinging in a hammock or on a swing:** Gently swaying in a hammock can provide a rhythmic and soothing motion that can help calm your nerves.

→ **Rocking in a rocking chair:** Sitting in a rocking chair or recliner that rocks slowly back and forth can have a relaxing effect on your body.

→ **Walking or hiking:** Taking a leisurely walk in nature or going for a hike allows you to experience the repetitive movement of walking while enjoying the outdoors.

→ **Swimming:** The rhythmic motion of swimming can be very calming. The water's resistance and buoyancy provide a soothing experience.

→ **Pacing:** Walking back and forth in a quiet room or a serene outdoor space can provide a repetitive, calming movement.

→ **Bouncing on an exercise ball:** Gently bouncing on an exercise ball can provide a subtle rocking motion that helps relieve tension.

→ **Swaying with music:** Swaying to slow, soothing music can be a natural way to experience calming movement.

→ **Knitting or crocheting:** Engaging in these crafts involves repetitive hand movements that can be meditative and calming. Some of my clients enjoy using craft kits for felting or even kits to paint role-playing game miniatures.

→ **Gardening:** Tasks like raking, digging, or planting involve repetitive movements and can be a therapeutic way to connect with nature.

→ **Playing a musical instrument:** Playing instruments like the piano, guitar, or drums involves coordinated and repetitive movements that can be relaxing. Even if you're not a drummer, tapping your pen on the table works just as well for calming.

→ **Kneading dough:** Whether it's bread dough in the kitchen, or Play-Doh at the table, taking a lump and massaging it through your hands is a repetitive movement experience that is predictable and soothing.

If you are looking to move more without structured exercise, one of my favorite resources for this is the work of Katy Bowman. She is the author of *Move Your DNA* and her concept of a "movement diet" is smart, fun, and easy to implement.[20] Incorporation of planned, intentional movement is an easy way to not only feel better but also to tame tics.

Step 6: Explore Your Sensory System.

"His sleep is really bad. He tells me he has restless legs all the time that bug him when he is trying to fall asleep. Sometimes I rub his legs and it helps a bit," the mother of eleven-year-old David told me.

"Whenever we go to any place with crowds at all, even say, the grocery store, her tics flare up immediately. She says that the noises make her annoyed, and she definitely gets more irritable. What can I do?" says the father of thirteen-year-old Anna.

"On days when I have to go into the office, it seems like my tics get worse. When I sit down at my desk and start working, that's when I notice it. I don't know why. Is it the fluorescent lights, maybe? It seems like sitting under them makes my tics worse," twenty-five-year-old Joel asked me.

You may have noticed patterns around your sensory system seemingly linked to how frequent or severe your (or your child's) tics are. You may have written this off, thinking that there was not much to be done, or tried some random different things, like throwing pasta against the wall to see "what sticks."

Or you may have dismissed sensory differences as not being related to tics or been unaware that they could be subtly (or not so subtly) influencing tics. As we will see, the sensory systems of people with tic disorders tend to be different from the general population, and sensory inputs can definitely impact tics. Let's explore this area of tic management to take advantage of the resources and strategies available.

As an occupational therapist, I am passionate about looking at life through a sensory lens. Just like we have body systems operating in the background without our conscious awareness, our sensory system is always "on." You can liken this system to a radar continuously scanning our environments (both inner and outer) to determine whether or not we are safe. The only problem with this is that sometimes the messages can be faulty; they can be too intense and cause interference, or they can be fuzzy, not allowing us to fully experience our world.

In Tourette Syndrome and tic disorders, there are often differences in the ways that sensory information is processed and integrated.[21] What is commonly observed and indicated is that people with Tourette Syndrome tend to have a hypersensitive threshold to sensory inputs as opposed to people without tic disorders. Some of these sensitivities involve atypical responses to heat and even a tendency for restless leg syndrome.[22]

Researchers have even found that adults with Tourette Syndrome have shown increased neural activity in areas associated with sensory feedback.[23] You have probably already noticed another sensory phenomenon: mirroring. This is when you imitate (or mirror) another person's tics, whether they are observed in person or even on video. People with tics of all ages also often report a strong feeling of needing to "get energy out" when they feel the need to tic). Interestingly, children and adults with anxiety (a common co-occurring condition) also tend to demonstrate increased body-based symptoms (anxiety) and awareness of heartbeat as opposed to others without anxiety.[24]

As a caregiver of someone with a tic disorder (or someone with a tic disorder yourself), it is very likely that you have seen how some of these sensory differences make coping with tics harder. Let's explore some of the sensory areas that tend to have big impacts and identify methods and tools that can support better tic management on our journey.

Auditory System: When Sounds Can Be a Tic Trigger

If you live with tics, or someone in your family does, you may know this all too well: sounds can be a huge tic trigger. Whether it is the sudden dropping of ice in the ice maker triggering tics or kids chatting and whispering in the classroom, for some people the noises in our environment can greatly impact tic severity.

When you know, or suspect, that sounds in your environment are contributing to tics, what can you do? Let's dive into practical things that you can implement today that may reduce auditory triggers.

If sounds in your environment are triggering tics, here are some of my recommendations for things you can try out today. Remember to approach these tools as an investigation into what your sensory system responds to. What works for one person will not necessarily be beneficial for another.

Colored Noise for Sleep or Calm

Some of the recommendations here are to dampen noises in our environment that can be exacerbating to tics. However, even deliberately "adding in" sounds may improve mood, sleep, and emotional responses. You may have heard of white noise, and may already use a white noise app to try to reduce some of the sounds in your environment while trying to sleep or relax. But did you know that there is a whole spectrum of colored noise?[25]

White noise is the most commonly referenced type of noise for calm, and there are many white noise apps and machines on the market. White noise can sound similar to a static noise in between channels on a TV. Many people listen to this type to fall asleep. Pink noise is considered to be a lower pitch than white noise, and research has shown that listening to it while trying to fall asleep can reduce sleep latency (the amount of time it takes to fall asleep)[26]. Brown noise, also sometimes called red noise, has a higher intensity at lower frequencies, even more so than white and pink noise. Some say it sounds like a low roar. I recommend trying out these various types of noise and not just as an adjunct to your sleep routine (although they may help). You can also use these noises in the background when working, studying, or when you are in an area with noise you cannot avoid (say when young kids are playing around you in the living room).

Another type of noise or sounds that can be helpful for calming include Autonomous Sensory Meridian Response (ASMR). You may have seen the YouTube channels that display calming videos of role-playing whispers, crinkling sounds, and cutting sounds that are increasing in popularity. Although there is limited research on ASMR, there is some evidence that it can help promote improved sleep quality.[27] Anecdotally, I have had clients (mainly teens) that find listening to ASMR videos helps them focus on tasks and regain calm after a distressing emotional situation or tic flareup.

Binaural Beats

Have you ever heard of binaural beats? They are a type of auditory stimulation usually presented with music. The concept of binaural beats is this: when two tones of similar frequencies are presented in each ear, the brain responds by perceiving a third tone, known as a binaural beat, which is said to be the difference in frequency between the two tones.

Binaural beat technology is marketed as a self-improvement tool and is reported to be able to reduce stress, improve anxiety, and increase focus and concentration. It is reported that binaural beat technology works by promoting changes in brain wave activity. A recent pilot study reported that use of binaural beats for a three-week period resulted in reduced perceived stress as well as a reduction in insomnia.[28]

If you'd like to try binaural beats yourself, you can find many free videos using binaural beat soundtracks on YouTube, although I can't vouch for how effective they are. I would recommend wearing stereo headphones while listening, listening for a minimum of fifteen minutes per day, and ensuring that you are doing a calming (as opposed to stimulating) activity while listening. I have personally used the Brainwave: 35 Binaural Series app and like the offerings of beat selections, from alerting and focus to tracks that promote calm and relaxation.

How about the sounds that are annoying, painful, and dysregulating that you cannot avoid? What can we do about that? There are times when you know you are going to want to protect your nervous system from excessive or distressing sounds, as they may trigger tics. Times such as being in a classroom with hard furniture that seems to let sounds bounce around or being together at a large family gathering with a lot of talking. If you have sensory sensitivity at all, being in these environments can be challenging.

One of my favorite tools for auditory sensitivity are called Loop earplugs. They are small, unobtrusive earplugs that can be worn by people of any age, even small children. They use acoustic resonance and noise filtering to allow sounds to continue to be heard clearly, just at a reduced volume. I have had many clients wear and benefit from them, and I wear them myself.

There are also additional therapies that can help with auditory sensitivity. One of them is called the Safe and Sound Protocol. This is a listening therapy that is designed to reduce stress and auditory sensitivity while enhancing social engagement and resilience.[29] This therapy is simple and can be relatively quick to complete. It essentially involves listening to filtered music, and the core of the program is only five hours long. It works by using specially filtered music to train the brain to attend to frequencies of human speech associated with safety, and in doing so stimulates the vagus nerve, strengthening the parasympathetic (or rest and digest) nervous system. As a provider of the Safe and Sound Protocol, you can find out more about it on my website.

Visual System: When Sights Can Be a Trigger

Having eye blinking tics is a common issue for many people. I often hear parents tell me that their child tics more when watching TV or being in front of the computer. When the child hears this they typically vehemently deny this, thinking I am going to recommend a ban on electronics for the sake of improving tics. Rest assured that I am not. Computers and technology are an integral part of our lives. So what can we do about the concern with eye tic exacerbation?

The first easy step to take is to reduce blue light and visual eye strain. For those of you that know about blue light, you are aware of its influence on energy or arousal state. If you are not familiar with the concept of blue light, it is essentially a color of light on the spectrum of light colors that is composed of short, high amplitude waves and is often associated with the use of technology.

Many of us, children included, spend most of our time indoors where we are exposed to more blue light than ever thanks to LED (light-emitting diode) technology. All of our computer and laptop screens, flat-screen televisions, cell phones, and tablets use this LED technology with high amounts of blue light. Although blue light also comes from the sun, it is more concentrated when we are sitting near the source, such as our backlit screens. And because we often spend hours closely focusing on these screens, they have an effect on our eyes and brain.

Although the research is a bit lacking and so far does not directly confirm that blue light causes eye strain and fatigue, you may have noticed this anecdotally. It is also true that, when looking at screens, we tend to blink less, causing drier eyes. These two components (as well as the fast-moving images that cause our eyes to make continual, lightning-quick saccades) can contribute to eye tics, such as blinking and rolling. A great number of my clients and their parents (particularly children and teens) report that using LED screens is a trigger for eye tics. Let's identify the things we can do to reduce this eye strain to enable us to use screens with less tic triggers.

The most obvious and easiest intervention is to simply monitor and reduce screen time to determine your individual effects. Remember, in managing our tics, data is our friend that helps us in making decisions.

If using LED screens for longer durations is a nonnegotiable for you due to online school or work, don't forget to take breaks. Try the 20-20-20 rule: Every twenty minutes, look at something twenty feet away for at least twenty seconds. Look as far out in the horizon as you can (say looking out a window down the street to the farthest object you can see). Why is this helpful? It promotes more blinking as it takes you away from focusing on the screen, which may help with eye moisture. It also gives your eyes a change from focusing inward (convergence) to focusing outward (divergence) which reduces the strain on your eye muscles.

Consider filtering the blue light with blue-light blocking glasses. These are readily available and inexpensive to purchase online. Trial wearing them while on the computer and when using electronics in the few hours before bedtime.

Additional benefits of reduction of blue light or increased exposure to red light include better sleep. A recent study of adults with Tourette Syndrome indicated that using light therapy in combination with reduction of blue light promoted increased sleep satisfaction.[30] If you have difficulty with insomnia, another product to try is called the Re-Timer. These specialized light-therapy glasses can help improve you or your child's circadian rhythm for improved sleep quality and onset.[31]

If you choose not to wear blue light glasses, or are simply looking for another alternative, I highly recommend the website f.lux. Here you can download free software for use on your Mac or Windows computer that automatically adapts the color of the display, making the color spectrum warm at night and like sunlight during the day for optimizing your eye's exposure to light. Other computers may have coloring filters built in and are available under settings.

Olfactory System: Smelling Our Way to Calm

You may have noticed that smell can promote very strong reactions in our bodies. From the soothing and compelling smell of your favorite meal or dessert (there is a reason realtors bake cookies at open houses) to the visceral smell of trash that needs our attention, smells impact us more than we realize. For starters, smells that we are sensitive to (such as an overwhelming candle or perfume) take up valuable attention and brain space as we struggle to regulate. And smells that are energizing (like peppermint or rosemary) can help us feel more productive. There are some smells that remind us of home and comfort (like the smell of your sweet old dog when he comes up to nudge you to pet him).

In my work with my clients, we often use smells as a way to regulate emotions. This, in tandem, can have a calming effect on tics and can help a person during a "tic attack" or an acute tic flareup. You can make your own scent vials using a cotton ball saturated with essential oils in a small glass container. Before you begin, a word of caution: some people are very sensitive to fragrance and can be allergic to certain scents. Do not use any essential oil until you are sure how it will affect you or your child. Here are my recommendations for scents you can try to create your own scent kit:

1. **Alerting:** Peppermint, rosemary, citrus (lemon, grapefruit, or lime), coffee beans. If you don't want to use oils, you can try to peel a citrus fruit to smell the natural aroma of the oils or suck on a peppermint candy. When working on homework or a project, you can prime your ability to focus by using the same scent each time before you begin.

2. **Calming:** Lavender, jasmine, vanilla, apple. You can create your own stovetop potpourri by simmering apple slices, vanilla beans, and more if you'd like to keep things even more natural. And as a bonus, your entire family can benefit from the aroma.

3. **Calming:** Familiar scents that remind us of home can be very soothing, particularly for children. You can keep a blanket or hoodie near (or wear one) that has the smell of home or lay on the floor next to your dog, nuzzling into his fur. I recommend bringing your own light blanket when traveling as well to allow you to bring these comforting scents when away and in a hotel room that may smell different or like cleaning products.

Touch and Proprioception: The Pressure That Soothes

Proprioception is the sense of body position, self-movement, and pressure. Although this sense may not be widely known, you can grasp the calming sensation of proprioception (and deep pressure) when getting a massage, a bear hug, or feeling the support of your favorite recliner cushioning your body. It can be linked and connected with touch, as many proprioceptive inputs are also experienced alongside it. Proprioception also helps our brain register where our body is in space so that we can move with coordination and balance (think about knowing where your feet are when sitting in a chair to be able to stand up with fluid motion).

Being close in proximity to other people (say in a tight crowd or when changing classes in a hallway) also activates the sense of proprioception, along with touch and sound (and even smell, if close enough). People who experience tics may notice that they can be triggered by these types of sensory inputs in small spaces. And as we've seen, people with OCD and Tourette Syndrome report heightened sensory sensitivity or intolerances to external sensory inputs.

Although touch (particularly light touch) can sometimes be alerting and contribute to tic exacerbation, deep pressure proprioceptive inputs are among the most calming. We can use these inputs as tools to influence tic severity and frequency. There is a significant body of research demonstrating the use of deep pressure touch to calm anxiety and improve sleep in people with and without autism spectrum disorder (ASD), anxiety, as well as ADHD.[32] [33]

What are the best ways to use deep pressure? Here is what I recommend to my clients:

1. Compression is a great way to calm the body that is lightweight, portable, and not hot. For active children who need to move, I typically recommend that they try a lycra body sock. This is essentially a stretchy lycra pouch that compresses the body gently during movements. They can jump, crawl, and generally play inside. Another option for sleep is to use compression sheets on the bed. Available in several sizes, these are a good choice over weighted blankets for summer or hot climates. Another benefit is they tend to be helpful with restless legs and trouble falling asleep.

2. Along with a compression sheet, some people prefer a weighted blanket or lap pad. This is a blanket that has weighted material sewn in to increase the weight and distribute it evenly over the body. The pressure of the blanket all over the body has a calming effect. A recent study also indicated that using a weighted blanket was associated with a pre-sleep increase in the body's natural melatonin production. It is not suggested to use a weighted blanket above 10 to 12 percent of your body weight. There are many brands available, however, I have had

a good experience with blankets with sewn-in glass beads, though you will need a washable cover.

3. Have someone roll a yoga ball over your body when lying on your stomach. The even, deep pressure on your back, arms, and legs can be relaxing and calming. Avoid the neck and head, and ask the person if the level of pressure should be decreased or increased.

4. Massage is another way to relieve pain and provide deep tactile pressure for calming. It can be tricky to use massage on yourself if you don't have a helper. Massage guns can be beneficial for pain reduction on sore muscles from motor tics and have various heads that can allow for broader or more targeted massage. They can be powerful, however, and I don't recommend them for children. For kids, massage rollers (either smooth or with spiky acupressure points) can be fun to use themselves and offer distraction and pain relief. Bonus points if you get your child to give you a foot or back massage!

Can sensory inputs help during a tic attack? They sure do! Here are some of the top things I recommend my clients do (and not do) to help them manage a tic attack:

Do's:

→ Make sure the person is safe (ex: motor tics aren't causing physical harm).

→ Shift focus of attention from inside to outside of body with distraction (can use grounding techniques, etc.).

→ Help the person manage anxiety with familiar coping techniques they have practiced and used before.

→ Encourage active sensory inputs that will provide distraction and not frustration (singing to favorite music, blowing bubbles and popping them, playing with kinetic sand).

→ Offer participation in rhythmic activity (dribbling a ball or tossing from hand to hand, rocking on a yoga ball, rocking on a glider or swing, using kazoo to hum a song with a beat or pattern, guided seated weight shifting back and forth with feet on a balance board or a wiggle cushion).

→ Use tactile and emotional benefit of pets (petting animal, brushing).

Don'ts:

→ Intervene in the process, actively trying to soothe the tics away and giving them undue attention and focus.

→ Comment about how a person feels or the tics themselves: "How do you feel? Are you okay?"

→ Encourage breathing if it is not helpful for them (can be a trigger for frustration or make tics worse).

Tic attacks can be scary and upsetting. But know that they will eventually subside and the more resilient you can make your nervous system, the more quickly you can return to feeling better emotionally after the tics are over.

Step 7: Improve Emotional Regulation.

For some parents I meet with, they tell me, "The tics are the least of our problems. What's even more troublesome are the behaviors my child has and the meltdowns that happen at least once a week!" Does that sound familiar to you?

Having problems with emotional regulation can make life difficult—to put it mildly! I've had parents tell me that their child's frequent dysregulation is making them unhappy and their home a place they dread to be. They've told me that the climate of the household can completely change in a matter of minutes. When I work with children who have challenges with emotional regulation, they are often aware of this and will report that they wish they didn't feel overwhelmed or as angry as much as they do.

Even if anger or rage seems to come out of nowhere with no direct outer alarm signs, if we look deeper we can see that there tend to be subtle ways our bodies and brains communicate with us and others. Red alert, things are about to get crazy! If we aren't attuned to these signs or have never learned what they are, we won't be able to intervene with enough time in the dysregulation arc to be effective.

Wait, dysregulation arc? There's an arc? Oh yes, there is, even if we don't know about it. Our brains are always scanning the environment for potential danger at an unconscious level of awareness called neuroception.

Here's how this arc of dysregulation plays out:

1. Your child is calm and at baseline level of nervous system arousal.
2. A known or unknown trigger of varying intensity occurs.

3. Sympathetic nervous system (gas pedal) is depressed, and escalation begins.
4. Escalation continues into dysregulation (top of arc).
5. Calming begins. (Brake pedal is activated; arc is trending downward.)
6. Return to baseline level of nervous system arousal.

The Arc of Dysregulation

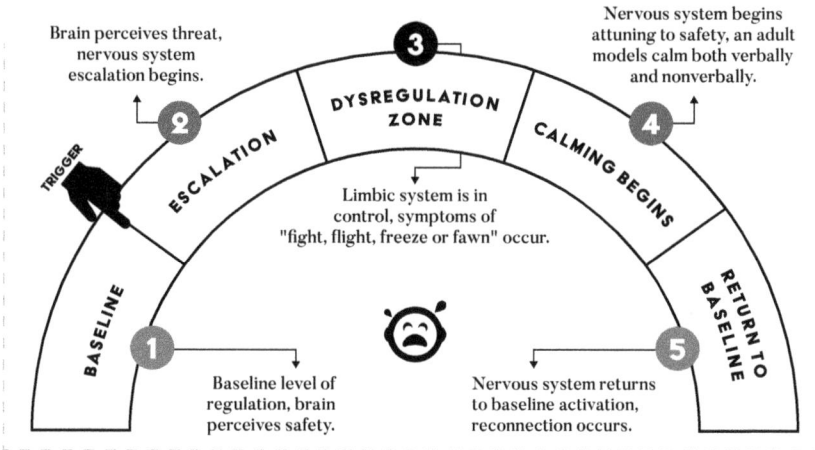

Where Do We Start?

Before we discuss where to begin with helping your child with emotional regulation, we need to visit the term self-regulation. Self-regulation is essentially a set of learned skills that enable a person to recognize and respond to emotions and situations with appropriate behaviors and actions. Sometimes, we try to put the cart before the horse and try to teach independent skills before children are developmentally ready. This can lead to frustration for all involved. It is also key to know that children and teens with ADHD tend to be behind their peers in the areas of emotional maturity and the skills of executive functioning (problem solving, time management, planning), even if they have other areas in which they excel. Also, some behaviors with emotional regulation can be related to expressions of anxiety.

Here's a handy chart that summarizes the age ranges expected for self-regulation skills. Keep in mind this is based on neurotypical functioning, and your child may or may not meet these milestones at the same time, or they may not be applicable for your child. These skills can be fluid, and they don't always fit neatly into a specific age range. The point here is to give you a reference point for what you might be able to expect from a developmental perspective.

Emotional Regulation Skills By Age

Birth to 2	→ Caregiver can model coping with emotions → Co-regulation essential for learning and achieving regulation → Adults begin to label and → identify emotions → Adults create a predictable routine for safety
Age 3-5	→ Caregiver can model coping with emotions (across all ages) → Co-regulation essential for learning and achieving regulation (across all ages) → Child begins to label and → identify emotions in self and others with assistance → Adults create a predictable routine for safety (across all ages) → Adults can model simple problem-solving language and strategies → Begins to demonstrate empathy for others

Age 5-8	→ Emotional vocabulary expands
	→ Self-awareness begins
	→ Beginning of perspective taking with assistance
	→ Can participate in adult-led problem-solving strategies
	→ Beginning of inhibitory control (ex: ability to wait)
	→ Empathy grows with modeling
	→ Use coping skills with support
Age 9-11	→ All skills listed previously with ability to expand independence in conflict management with support
	→ Increased ability to independently identify emotions in self and others
	→ Ability to use inhibitory control grows (being able to delay gratification to complete less-preferred task before preferred with support)
	→ Greater participation in problem solving with others
	→ Growth in assertiveness to identify boundaries with others
	→ Use coping skills with support
Age 12-14	→ Improved ability to self-reflect and greater self-knowledge
	→ Ability to understand nuances in emotion
	→ Increased ability to use problem-solving skills with greater independence
	→ Continued growth in navigating peer relationships
	→ Growth in inhibitory control to complete daily activities
	→ Use coping skills with greater independence
Age 15-18	→ All skills listed previously
	→ Improved resilience (bouncing back from challenging event)
	→ Uses coping skills with greater independence
	→ Benefits from a mix of guided decision making and independence with logical consequences
	→ Greater ability to generalize perspective taking
	→ Improves in interpersonal communication (listening to others, giving and receiving feedback, etc.)
	→ Growth in self-awareness and social awareness

Once you know when developmental self-regulation skills emerge (in general), you can get started in helping your child learn and apply the skills they need. But first, let's learn about what actually happens when a child or teen becomes dysregulated using the framework of the arc.

Baseline Level

What it looks like:

Physical

→ Pulse and pupil dilation is normal

→ Breaths per minute are normal

→ Muscle tension is normal

→ Movements are normal

→ Responses to sensory inputs are normal

Emotional and Cognitive

→ Able to engage in activity such as learning and interacting with others

→ Able to choose and use coping strategies (for practice, learning, and generalization) independently or with some help

→ Able to use higher-level thinking and has increased tolerance for challenge and problem solving

Dysregulation Is Triggered (Brain Senses Danger)

What it looks like:

Physical

→ Pulse and pupil dilation may change, pulse may increase to reflect greater sympathetic activation, and pupils may dilate slightly

→ Breaths per minute may increase slightly above normal baseline

→ Tension on muscles starts to increase (think, shoulders begin to get elevated, arms and legs may move inward for protection and ready response due to sympathetic activation)

→ Movement speed may increase or decrease, reflecting body's readiness to either fight, flight, or freeze

→ May exhibit exaggerated responses to inputs that are tolerated differently when not in a sympathetically activated state (noises seem louder, smells are harder to tolerate, people being closer in proximity is more agitating)

→ Voice becomes louder

Emotional and Cognitive

→ Unable to access problem solving and rational areas of the brain

→ Emotionally reactive and over-responsive

→ Attempts to calm not usually effective

→ May respond to safe people with offensive statements, insults, or physical attacks due to brain's perception of danger

Rage and Dysregulation Peaks

Above symptoms, with greater intensity

De-escalation, Calming

What it looks like:

Physical

→ Pulse and pupil dilation slowly return to normal

→ Breaths per minute slowly return to normal

→ Muscle tension slowly returns to normal

→ Movements slow

→ Responses to sensory inputs slowly return to normal

Emotional and Cognitive

→ Sometimes expresses embarrassment
for reactions

→ Attempts reconnection with safe people
(apologizing, coming near or needing proximity
and closeness)

→ Attempts resolution if able

Return to Baseline

In my work with families, one of the things I always help them understand as being crucial is using the right tool or strategy at the right
time. Unfortunately, once a child is at the peak of the dysregulation
arc, most tools will not be very effective. You may have observed this
yourself. Why is that?

Once we move to the top of the arc and are dysregulated, the
brain's job moves from detecting threat to preserving the body's safety.
This is when the older part of our brain, the limbic system, is most
activated. Within the limbic system are brain areas you may have
heard of, including the amygdala, hippocampus, and cingulate gyrus.
When the brain is on a protection mission, it is very difficult to engage
other parts of the brain that help us with rational thinking, choice,
and using learned skills (the prefrontal cortex). Biologically, they just
aren't as important in helping us survive in a crisis.

It is only after the limbic system becomes less activated that we
can actually begin to use the tools, strategies, and skills we know. Less
activation of the limbic system means that the brain can now use the

prefrontal cortex where we can decide if we should change course, try a familiar strategy, or ask for help. If your child is younger, this may be the point where they can actually respond to your coaching and scaffolding of skills.

How To Improve and Manage Emotional Regulation Challenges

If your child's rage or frequent dysregulation is wreaking havoc in your family, what are the steps you need to take? Here is the process I recommend to my clients.

1: Fill Up Your Own Cup First—All the Way!

Most people don't realize how little capacity they have for stress due to the continual inundating challenges that they face daily. I don't need to remind you of the way the pit of your stomach feels when you get that unexpected bill, the email from the teacher that your child is having problems behaving in class, the project at work that must be done immediately, and so on. As these things tend to be out of our control, we keep moving through life tackling the next thing. Over time, our own nervous system's resilience decreases, making us less able to respond to challenges without distress. Even if you feel you are handling life's challenges well, there is a good chance that you may be experiencing hidden symptoms of stress's toll. These include having high cortisol levels, elevated blood pressure, or symptoms of inflammation. You may also be aware of your own symptoms of anxiety, irritability, or depression.

The first thing to do, before addressing your child's anxiety or dysregulation, is to equip yourself with tools that work for you. In order for you to be able to manage your child's symptoms effectively, you must first "put on your own air mask." This is an essential step. Have you even tried to calm someone down when you are scared or upset yourself? Our emotions are heavily influenced by those around us, and in fact we take emotional cues from others' unspoken body language and facial expressions. I will be making recommendations in this section on tools to help your child cope with rage, anxiety, and dysregulation. I highly recommend that you also explore the tools and strategies presented here and create your own "Regulation Toolkit" to implement on a regular basis. It will make it so much easier to help your child when you are operating from a place of regulation and calm yourself. Remember, we are not looking for perfection here.

When working with families, I often employ tools for the parent or caregiver first, ranging from use of an auditory vagus nerve stimulation program, heart-rate variability training, or counseling if needed.

2: Use Co-Regulation, No Matter Your Child's Age.

Co-regulation is one of the latest buzzwords in the therapy space. But although this might seem new to you, you've been participating in co-regulation activities since your child was born.

One of the most common ways we co-regulate is to pick up, rock, and soothe a crying infant. We intuitively know that babies do not have the ability to calm themselves without assistance, and we also know that their crying is the only way they have to communicate their needs. As we talked about, one of the cool things about the nervous system and mirror neuron network is that, even without saying a word, we can lend another person our calm (or our distress). We even take advantage of this phenomenon as adults when we ask for a hug from our spouse after a hard day or stressful event, or we call a friend to vent about something that upset us, and we noticeably feel better.

So why do we believe after the toddler years that our children are completely ready to regulate on their own (self-regulate)? Although the topic of co-regulation can be a whole book (and there are many), to simplify this process, you can try the following to help your child or teen when they are distressed and need your calm, experienced nervous system (this is the top of the arc):

→ Provide proximity. Staying near your child when they are upset provides their nervous system with cues of safety.

→ Rather than matching their level of arousal (voice, body, and movements) choose to speak in a slow, neutral tone.

→ Intentionally move into low and slow breathing, but do not ask or require your child to imitate you. This serves to calm your body and give you more emotional bandwidth and also models for your child how breath can be used to de-escalate an emotional state. Every time you practice doing this, you get better and better at responding this way in the moment. You may also find that your child's pace of breathing starts to mimic yours.

→ Use reflective statements in your communication. ("It sounds like you are saying…, is that right?") This does not mean that you have to approve or agree with the request, simply that you are demonstrating that you understand.

If this is an area that you would like to explore more (and the concept of self-regulation in general), I highly recommend the book by Robyn Gobbel, *Raising Kids with Big Baffling Behaviors.*[34]

Having an understanding of self-regulation in yourself and your child will go miles in helping you help them cope with tics and the challenges they bring. You can do it! But again, if you are looking for more help and someone to walk you through your individual situation, I help families like yours every day in my work, and would love to help you!

3: Ensure Expectations and Demands Are Appropriate, Break Down into Smaller Tasks as Needed.

The fastest way to emotional upset is to provide a task or demand that a child is not ready to meet without support. This could be a simple request such as, "Can you clean your room please?" or "Have you done all of your homework?" If you are noticing a pattern of tasks or activities that seem to be difficult for your child (and thus difficult for you), consider that they may not have the skills needed to intuitively break the task down into manageable pieces to make traction and complete the task. They may struggle with task endurance and inhibition to keep working at a task that is challenging. It may seem frustrating that your child is fully competent in other areas of life, but we have to remember that inner motivation plays a huge role in our effectiveness. Until they are more motivated and the activity is easier, we need to scaffold the task.

Imagine you've got a messy car and take it to the car wash. Do you have a plan or sequence that you follow automatically? Do you start vacuuming before you throw away the trash and put away small items?

If you did, it would make the task much harder (having to maneuver the vacuum around old water bottles, and you may even accidentally vacuum up the dollar bill in the cupholder). Do you have a vision in your head of how the car should look when you are done that helps you to know when to stop wiping, waxing, or vacuuming? Think about how hard this simple job would be if you did all the steps out of order, or if you did the whole task but didn't clean the bug-smeared windshield. Do you also have a good idea about how long the task should take and when it is appropriate to start it? (Not a good time to head to the carwash when you've got to leave for work in fifteen minutes.)

When we know an activity is hard for our child and may result in a meltdown, one way to help is to create a step-by-step plan (in writing or using visuals). Then they can complete each part, knowing exactly where they stand and how many small subtasks they have left to do. This is naturally more reassuring and will also help them build the skills they need to eventually complete other tasks on their own using the same organizational steps.

We often forget as adults how we do this intuitively, but remember, there are whole professions dedicated to helping break up complex projects and get them done (project management)! By the way, if doing this seems overwhelming to you, occupational therapists are experts at this (we call it task analysis). More later on how to find a *great* occupational therapist to help you on your journey.

4: Frontload and Teach Tools.

As we've discussed how crucial the timing of de-escalation can be, know that we can use this to our advantage rather than being at the mercy of it in the middle of an outburst of emotion. When should you be introducing and practicing these skills? The answer is before an outburst of rage or dysregulation occurs and as frequently as possible. You can also be modeling using these techniques yourself so that your child can see that you use them in calm states to keep you feeling good and not always associated with times of stress. You can choose to have a weekly time to teach or review tools that you have chosen or that your child has learned in therapy. The key is doing it with consistency and regularity so that these tools can be generalized and will be useful in the moment. I usually teach my clients and families to link the teaching and review of techniques to something they already have scheduled, such as Friday night dinners, or even driving in the car to a place they go weekly.

Remember, this must always be done proactively when your child (and you) is in a calm, regulated state. It is not the time to try a new "play" in the middle of the game.

If the challenge is task completion, you can have your child rank which tasks are easiest for them and identify which ones they may need support in during the coming week. Doing this on a weekend before the tasks are required to be completed is always more productive.

5: Learn to Recognize Your Child's Place on the Arc.

Often we feel that rage attacks happen suddenly without warning (and sometimes they do). But with some insight and data, you can learn and look for patterns that will help you figure out some of your child's triggers. This will allow you to intervene before they reach the peak of the arc. If your child or teen is at an age where they have the emotional maturity and insight to participate in self-reflection, they can also be part of the process to look for patterns or reflect on them.

(Warning: This is not appropriate during a meltdown, or recently after, or when emotions are still running high.)

One tool that occupational therapists often use to help children understand this process is through interoception interventions. Interoception is our way of processing and interpreting the signals of our internal sensory system (heart rate, muscle tension, dry throat, etc.). Making the connection between subtle shifts in these signals can help your child know that their internal safety trigger has gone off, and they are trending toward a fight-flight-or-freeze response.

6: Introduce, Select, and (Proactively) Practice Preferred "Feel-Good" Tools.

Here are some of the actual tools and techniques I use with my clients and families in therapy for tics to create their own Regulation Toolkit. These are my favorite, tried-and-true sensory strategies.

Changing Temperatures for Calm

We often gravitate toward warm temperatures when stressed. Those can be helpful tools to add to your toolkit. However, I also find that some of my clients like to use cold modalities, and they can be especially helpful when you or your child is trending up the arc to full dysregulation.

Cold Temperature Tools:

→ Take an ice pack from the freezer and apply to back of neck, inside of wrists, and even middle of chest. It is important to note that the person themself should be in charge of how much cold and where and when to apply. What feels good to one person may be too cold or unpleasant to another.

→ Try an ice water dunk. You can fill a bowl with ice and water and immerse a body part you desire. Some people choose to put their whole face in for a few seconds (intense cold) and some people prefer a fingertip or hand in the water. This is very alerting but can help us move out of a state of fight-or-flight quickly, as our brains are forced to attend to the physical sensations first. You may have heard of the "mammalian diver reflex." This is a physiological response that automatically happens to air-breathing mammals when they have to hold their breath when diving into cold water. This survival instinct slows down our heart rate, helping us to reduce anxiety immediately.

Warm Temperature Tools:

→ Use a warming microwavable rice pack.
→ Use hand warmers (can be purchased at Dollar Tree in cold months).
→ Wear warming slippers for feet.
→ Take a warm bath.
→ Cover self with blanket warmed from the dryer.

Deep Pressure Strategies

We explored several of these strategies in the sensory section. Try them and select the ones (if any) that you want to add to your toolkit.

Breath Strategies

When I mention breath strategies, often my clients say to me, "My therapist already told me about that, it doesn't work for me." So why do I continue to recommend breathing techniques as a strategy for managing dysregulation and tics? There are many reasons, but one of them is that studies have shown that breathing can reduce the intensity of tics, and it does work for many people.[35]

Low and Slow Breathing

When people engage in breath techniques, they are often instructed to "take a deep breath." This is not helpful, as it often leads to overbreathing, actually increasing anxiety and dysregulation. When I coach people to use breath strategies, such as diaphragmatic breathing, I always emphasize the need to breathe slowly (around six breaths per minute) rather than deeply.

When people experience a sudden onset of anxiety, they can begin breathing more shallowly and quickly. When this happens, hyperventilation can occur, although it often doesn't look like it does in the movies and is more subtle. Hyperventilation can cause a decreased level of carbon dioxide in the blood, which can result in feeling dizzy, shaky, lightheaded, and more. These physical symptoms often exacerbate anxiety and make the person feel worse. Using "low and slow" breathing can help restore the balance of carbon dioxide to oxygen, making the person feel better physically and less anxious. Research shows that using this technique can result in a shift toward parasympathetic dominance (the "rest and digest" branch of our autonomic nervous system).[36]

How do you do "low and slow" breathing? It simply means that you practice a nasal inhale of a slow, comfortable breath with a focus on allowing it to move down into your belly. Exhale is usually done with an open mouth, allowing the belly to fall back down slowly. You can practice this by using a breath pacer (link to a free one can be found on my website under the free resources section). Another key to low and slow breathing is to ensure that your exhale is nearly twice as long as the inhale. I recommend a goal of five minutes per day. This is a great thing to practice in the evening before bed or even upon waking in the morning. For my pediatric clients, we often create a video of them breathing with good pacing using various video editing tools such as Loom that they can show to their family and guide the practice.

Some fun ways to practice this low and slow breathing include:

→ **Teddy bear breathing:** Placing a small stuffed animal of your choice on your belly, allow it to rise on the inhale (keep it slow and breathing down to the belly), then allow it to move down with the belly on the slow exhale, giving it a "ride."

→ **Blowing bubbles:** This is an engaging way for both kids and adults to practice "low and slow breathing." Inhale slowly through the nose, then exhale slowly through the mouth with the wand in front of you. Try to make a large bubble if you can.

→ **Word length breath:** Once you've determined a good tempo for your low and slow breaths, choose two long words that you can say in your mind as you breathe in and out. This will help you keep time and offer a distraction during the breath if needed. For instance: "Encyclopedia (in breath) Britannica (out breath)."

Physiological Sigh (a.k.a. Double Inhale)

I was first introduced to this simple but effective technique by neuroscientist and professor Andrew Huberman. Here's how you do it: Take two inhales through the nose (one big, one smaller) then one long exhale through the mouth until lungs empty. Repeat as needed.

Dr. Huberman claims that even just one physiologic sigh is the fastest way to bring about calm in real time, and my clients that have tried it confirm this (and I do too!)

Lateral Eye Movement

You may be familiar with the therapeutic intervention called EMDR (eye movement desensitization and reprocessing). This is often used in therapy to increase calm and help people process traumas.

Did you know that the psychologist who discovered this technique was taking a walk in the woods when she realized that the reflexive side-to-side eye movement that occurs with forward movement calmed her? Turns out this movement can suppress activation of the amygdala, reducing anxiety. You don't have to see an EMDR therapist to get some of the benefits of this technique. Here's how:

→ Engage in forward movement in your environment to initiate this reflexive side-to-side eye movement.
→ You can do this by running, walking, skating, or cycling.
→ Don't look at your phone while moving.
→ Try to sustain the movement continuously over a period of ten to twenty minutes.

→ You get a double benefit as forward movement shifts our "attentional flashlight" for tic management.

Progressive Muscle Relaxation

Progressive muscle relaxation (PMR) is the sequenced tensing and relaxing of muscles. This can be paired with an auditory track or video for pacing and cuing to move through the body. A benefit of PMR is that it can be used discretely anywhere. With my pediatric clients, we often create a PMR story that they can easily remember. I typically have them choose a theme that they like, and together we invent a story about each area they are tensing and relaxing so that they can remember it without help.

The contrast you feel between tightening and relaxing helps to alleviate muscle soreness and tension from tics as well as promoting a general feeling of relaxation. I often use this technique when my mind wanders to a stressful topic while driving.

7: Engage in Reconnection and Skill Building.

After an outburst of rage or emotional dysregulation, always end with reconnecting with your child. This reconnection can have many forms, such as sitting together on the couch, going on a walk together, or giving each other a hug. Your child needs to hear and experience (over and over again) that they are loved unconditionally. Experiencing emotional challenges does not impact their place in the family, and this knowledge helps to provide a solid foundation of psychological safety and maturity to enable growth. You already know this, or you wouldn't be reading this book.

Only after your child has securely returned to their baseline state of emotional regulation do we attempt teaching and skill building. That's the time when proactive problem solving can occur, making the next challenging episode easier.

I highly recommend Dr. Ross Greene's collaborative problem-solving approach. This evidence-based approach helps walk you through these necessary problem-solving steps, and what's more, his handouts for the process are completely free on his website at www.livesinthebalance.org.

Self-regulation is a skill set that takes a long time to develop, especially for kids and teens with tic disorders and co-occurring conditions. Be gentle with yourself (especially on those days when you feel like you are going to lose your mind!) You'll eventually come to learn techniques that will make life easier for both you and your child.

8: Improve Overall Nervous System Resilience.

For some of my clients, I recommend biofeedback as a way to tap into the body's built-in stress-relieving and coping mechanisms. Although there are a variety of types of biofeedback, including neuromuscular biofeedback, thermal biofeedback, and EEG neurofeedback, the type I recommend the most is heart-rate variability biofeedback (HRV). The reasons are simple: this type of biofeedback is widely available, easy, and motivating to do (even for children) and promotes inner resilience for better management of emotions and nervous system arousal.

Here's how it works: A person is instructed to breathe at a slow and low pace (how slow is based upon measurements of that person's resonance frequency, but typically between five to seven breaths per minute). While using a finger sensor, the chosen software calculates the heart-rate variability (essentially a marker of the resilience of the parasympathetic branch of our autonomic nervous system, sometimes known as "Rest and Digest") and feeds back information and visuals to help the person know how they are doing. Depending on the software you use, you could experience a tree growing, a car racing down a track, or a beautiful visual brighten and darken based upon how close you are to the optimal heart-rate variability target. As you train, over time you will experience an increase in your heart-rate variability metrics, which directly correlates with strengthening of the parasympathetic branch of your nervous system. This leads to greater internal calm, an increased emotional "buffer" for improved emotional regulation, as well as other health benefits for both kids and adults.

One of my favorite companies that provides direct-to-consumer heart-rate variability sensors and apps/games is called HeartMath (www.heartmath.com). You can order a sensor online and use the app to take baseline data and train in one day, without needing a prescription or medical professional to access.

Improving Impulse Control, Naturally

Another challenge for children and teens with Tourette Syndrome (and co-occurring ADHD) is delayed impulse control. Although counseling with techniques such as cognitive behavioral therapy can help your child learn strategies to prevent and cope with impulsivity and inhibition, this issue is often continually problematic. How can you work on inhibition from the inside out?

One of my recommendations for my clients is the use of a therapy modality called Interactive Metronome. This computer-based training system promotes decreases in impulsivity, greater focus and attention, and even gains in executive functioning skills. It works by teaching your child to use inner, neural timing to connect motor movements and auditory inputs with millisecond accuracy. This modality can be used by anyone from elite athletes looking for an edge with their motor skills to a child with poor attention, impulsivity, or delays in language skills.

Here's how it works: After an assessment of your child's coordination, timing, and ability to attend over time we create a treatment plan. The sessions consist of movements to an auditory beat (a metronome) that is measured to the millisecond. We often find that children and adults with ADHD or frequent impulsivity demonstrate movements that are ahead of the beat. Through practice and visuals/sounds that help the person improve, they learn to respond to the input with more control, less reactivity, and specific accuracy. These new skills translate to all sorts of improvements and can help a person benefit even more from the concepts they learn in traditional therapy.

In my practice, I combine Interactive Metronome training with the use of cognitive tools to help people of all ages reduce impulsivity and increase attention and inhibition. This intervention can even be done remotely when you receive your equipment for home use. Unlike heart-rate variability biofeedback, Interactive Metronome requires the coaching and assessment of a medical provider. If you are interested in this effective modality (or biofeedback) for yourself or your child, you can find out more about it on my website.

Step 8: Look for Food Sensitivities and Triggers.

Let's be clear on nutrition, diet, and food sensitivities. As an occupational therapist, I spent quite a bit of time in my school's cadaver lab learning all about anatomy and physiology. I learned about statistics, patient care, and kinesiology. I learned about the myriad of conditions that I would likely be treating, how they present, and how to determine best interventions for them. What did I learn absolutely nothing about? Nutrition! Despite the fact that the food we intake is literally building our bodies from the inside out, many professionals learn little, if anything, about nutrition in school (unless they are going to school to be a dietician). And what happens to things we don't know about? We tend to dismiss them. It is not surprising that most doctors will tell you that food and diet has nothing to do with tics. And your own lived experience may tell you the same. You may have experimented with different types of diets and noticed no changes in your mood or tics. And if so, that's absolutely okay.

As I mentioned before, I am not a nutritionist, and I do not have any expertise in assessing vitamin or mineral deficiencies. With that said, I do have years of experience in working with children, teens, and adults with tic disorders. Let me tell you a story about one of my recent clients and our discoveries about food intake and tic frequency/severity.

When I arrived for a session with my client, I asked how his tics were over the past week. "Terrible!" he said. "My cousins were visiting, and they were really flaring! I'm not sure why."

Hmmmm…. This is where we dig a little deeper and see if there are any patterns we can detect that are hiding right in front of us.

"Tell me about when your cousins were here. What was it like before they came? When they got here, what did you all do?"

"Oh! I love when they come to visit! I love them so much! We always make blanket pallets on the floor in the loft and watch movies together. We watched the whole *Star Wars* trilogy. It was awesome!"

Mom interjects: "Yes, and you had multiple bags of popcorn. Pretty much one bag a day. And I swear that eating popcorn makes you tic."

You can guess what happened. The teen rolled his eyes and exasperatedly groaned, "Mom, come on! It does not!"

Now at this point, I hadn't heard anyone tell me that popcorn can affect tics. I was definitely skeptical, however, I kept my comments to myself. I am an open-minded therapist, and I wanted to explore this and at least hear mom out. I asked her to elaborate on why she thought popcorn was a tic trigger for her son. She reported that she first made the connection a few years ago- that whenever they would have popcorn on family movie night soon after (and the day after as well) it seemed like his tics would increase significantly.

Upon hearing this, my client leapt up from his seat. "But mom, I don't want to give up popcorn. I won't!" Now she sighed and commented, "I know. It's your favorite." Have you ever met anyone who was a real popcorn person? That was this kid. And apparently she was minimizing the opportunities to have popcorn, and I was just now hearing about it.

I reassured my client that popcorn was going nowhere. I reaffirmed that he loved popcorn and it gave him joy when watching a movie. But I also reminded him that, as a "tic detective," it would be wise to look at this further to see if there was anything to it. I asked him if he would be willing to eat more popcorn, as an experiment. "Eat more popcorn?" he asked. "Yeah, I would!" Mom agreed, and we began the process of creating a very simple food diary/tracker. He would need to make sure he had popcorn at least a few times within the next two weeks, and we would look for changes in his tic patterns after he consumed it.

Fast forward two weeks later, and as soon as I entered the session, my client expressed, "Guess what? I found out that popcorn does make me tic! It actually made me tic a lot!" He showed me the data he had collected. And sure enough, several times, within thirty minutes of eating the popcorn, his tics increased dramatically. There was no denying a correlation. My next recommendations were for mom to have him assessed for potential food allergies or sensitivities if she felt that was warranted.

However, in the meantime, what did this mean for his tic management plan? The teen absolutely loved popcorn and refused to give it up. First, as you would predict, we brainstormed different types of popcorn that might affect him less (such as not eating microwave popcorn, changing brands of kernels, switching to organic/non-GMO, eating air popped popcorn, and using a different, less inflammatory oil). After these trials, it was still clear that, for whatever reason, popcorn (or corn) seemed to make his tics increase. We discussed this outcome and what he would do if his tics flared after the popcorn. We talked about when it would be okay to have the popcorn and when it might not, based on his preferences and needs. He decided that he would not want to eat popcorn with people he would be nervous to tic around or before a situation when increased tics would be inconvenient or embarrassing. He also decided, with his mother, that he didn't need to give up popcorn but would have it only when at home and when he was around people he felt safe to tic around in case his tics increased. They also decided that they would try some new, non-popcorn crunchy snacks to see if he liked something different that he could snack on during movies.

Like my client's mother, you may have some indications that certain foods or additives make your child's tics worse. What can you do about it? I would start first with a simple food diary/tracking sheet. You can find a free downloadable version on my website at www.helpfortics.com. When you have suspicions about food sensitivities being a tic trigger, the first thing you need to do is to narrow down what you are eating, when you are eating it, and what your tics are like. There are obviously many other variables, but I also do recommend that you add into the tracking sheet what you are doing and what your emotions were like at the time. Having information (lots of it) is the best way to see the small, underlying patterns that may be showing up continually, right under your nose.

If you suspect that you or your child have some vitamin or mineral deficiencies, or want to look into more info on a specific diet for your condition, I would recommend seeing a functional medicine doctor. There is an emerging area of research that demonstrates that specific ways of eating can impact mental health conditions. One example is the evidence that links a low carb/high fat diet with reduced anxiety.[37] I can personally absolutely vouch for this as someone with chronic anxiety; when I am eating less carbs my anxiety is noticeably reduced! We know that the more information we have about a person with tics, the easier it is to evaluate and connect the dots and have areas of focus for change. Using a holistic approach that combines addressing mental health, nervous system arousal, motivation, autonomy, and nutrition will go a long way in managing and improving tics for the long term.

Step 9: Prepare Your "Tic Talk" to Address Tics with Others.

So when you've got tics that can be disruptive in public, how do you live your life? What do you do when people are staring at you (or your child) and you just want to have a normal trip buying your groceries at Walmart? And when exactly should you bring up the topic of tics with your child and prepare them to explain what tics are to others?

The first thing I'd like to mention on this topic is that you don't have to tell others about your tics if you don't want to. This is a highly personal journey, and for some people tics are mild or can be suppressed in public. Friends, teachers, or colleagues may not know that someone has a tic disorder. If this is you (or your child), don't feel that it is necessary to reveal that you have tics. But if you've got loud vocal tics, or repetitive motor tics that often occur in public places, you may want to read on.

The Elephant in the Room

Why might you want to create your own "tic talk" or your way of explaining your tics to someone? For starters, it can get very annoying very quickly to have people asking over and over, "Are you okay?" or handing you a tissue when they hear you sniffing. When you can matter-of-factly explain that you have tics, nothing is wrong, and that they can ignore them, it takes their concern (and comments) out of the situation. Additionally, in the era of COVID, you may get side eyes from people if you have a frequent coughing tic in an enclosed space, such as on the middle seat in a crowded airplane. Telling your seatmate that you are actually not sick but may have a coughing tic can go a long way in allowing you to enjoy your flight without hostility from your neighbor.

And this is a key point: you don't tell people about your tics to ease their concerns but rather to allow you to feel at ease wherever you are if you think your tics might interfere.

A Hidden Disorder

Because many people have never been around someone with tics (or they don't think they have), they may not know what a tic looks like. This is in part because so many stereotypes in the media exist and what people think they know about tics is that they involve screaming obscenities. So when you or your child has a sniffing tic or a tongue-sticking-out tic, they don't understand it. Once people understand that these movements and sounds are involuntary, they typically respond with compassion—or at least stop asking about them.

Here's a way I advise my clients, whether they are adults, children, or teens, to talk to their peers or coworkers about tics:

Peer: "Why are you making that weird face so much?"

Person with tics: "It's just an automatic thing I do sometimes; it's called a tic. I have other ones occasionally too. You can just ignore it."

Peer: "Oh, okay."

And that's it. Not very complicated in most cases, and that usually resolves the other person's curiosity. If your child is being bullied or harassed, that's another story that involves addressing other parents or school administration.

Two other ways to address and bring tics to the forefront include having a Youth Ambassador talk with your child's class and having your child read a book about tics (if they choose to). Acknowledging your tics can go a long way in making you feel at ease wherever you are, and it gets so much easier to do this over time.

Step 10: Initiate Plan for Support at School or Work.

If you have a school-age child or teen, you may be worried about how they will cope with tics at school. You may have noticed that their tics can often seem to "explode" at the end of a school day. Helping your child with homework may be the hardest (and most dreaded) part of your day. Does your child need extra support at school? What support tools are available, and how do we access them?

You may have heard people talk about something called an IEP or a 504? What are those, and does my child need one? An IEP (or Individualized Education Plan) or a 504 (504 Plan, which comes from Section 504 of the Rehabilitation Act) are both tools that can be necessary for your child or teen to be successful in school. One caveat here: I do not recommend that either of these tools be provided to any and all students just because they have a diagnosis of a tic disorder. As you will learn, your child also needs to meet eligibility criteria beyond having a qualifying diagnosis and also has to demonstrate an educational need. Not sure which one might be needed, if at all?

Let's begin with the basics of an IEP. Before I became an occupational therapist, I was a special education teacher, and I have experience with both IEPs and 504 Plans from the perspective of both a teacher and therapist.

Individualized Education Plan (IEP)

What: An IEP stands for Individualized Education Plan. It is a document created for students with disabilities who require special education services in the United States and is an educational plan to address a person's needs related to learning to ensure equal access to education. The IEP is developed collaboratively by a team that includes the student's parents or guardians, teachers, special education professionals, and other relevant individuals.

The purpose of an IEP is to outline the specific educational goals and objectives for the student, as well as the specialized instruction and support services they will receive to help them meet those goals. It is tailored to the unique needs of each student and is reviewed and updated annually.

In order to qualify for an IEP under the Individuals with Disabilities Education Act (IDEA), a child's school performance must be "adversely affected" by a disability in one of thirteen categories:

→ Autism spectrum disorder
→ Blindness
→ Deafness
→ Emotional disturbance
→ Hearing impairment
→ Intellectual disability
→ Multiple disabilities
→ Orthopedic impairment
→ Other health impairment
→ Specific learning disability
→ Speech or language impairment
→ Traumatic brain injury
→ Visual impairment

If your child is struggling at school primarily due to a tic disorder, and does not have any other disability, they may qualify under the category of "other health impairment." This is also a common category for students who are struggling in school related to symptoms of ADHD, OCD, or Tourette Syndrome.

Who: A student with a diagnosis falling within the thirteen IDEA qualifying categories who demonstrates need based upon an educational evaluation performed by a multidisciplinary team. An IEP is for school-age children only, within the age range of three to twenty-two years old. Your school team may also use what is called a MTSS team (multi-tiered system of supports) where the education team uses interventions prior to testing for problem solving and decision-making to help the student.

Why: A student would benefit from an IEP if they are demonstrating difficulty with accessing learning in the school setting. This could mean that they are having difficulty with the academic content or that they have a behavioral or social-emotional challenge that makes learning difficult. This is important to note because IEP teams may often remark that a student doesn't need an IEP because they are passing all of their classes. Often, children and teens can have co-occurring executive functioning delays, language delays, anxiety, or intrusive thoughts. These delays or difficulties can make it hard for them to show what they know, stay organized enough to turn in assignments, and make sure they are completed on time. We also know that having difficulties with social communication and inhibition are often related to Tourette Syndrome, and many educators and teams are unaware of this.

How: Your best bet is to reach out to your child's school psychologist. The role of a school psychologist is to know education law and legalities, and they are often the lead or point of contact for a school assessment team. They can often provide you with further information about how to begin the process of determining if your child needs (or qualifies for) a 504 plan or IEP.

Now let's contrast a 504 plan to an IEP as it relates to students with tic disorders.

504 Plan

What: A 504 plan differs from an IEP in that it outlines accommodations and support services for students with disabilities who require assistance to fully participate in their education. It is named after Section 504 of the Rehabilitation Act of 1973, which prohibits discrimination based on disability in programs and activities that receive federal funding.

The purpose of a 504 Plan is to ensure that students with disabilities have equal access to education and are provided with necessary accommodations and modifications. It covers a wide range of disabilities, including but not limited to physical, medical, learning, and attention-related conditions. As you'll notice, however, the goal of a 504 is to allow *access to education* and is not a type of educational programming or intervention plan based upon learning or behavioral needs.

Why: Your child or teen may need a 504 if they have not documented an educational need that meets criteria for an IEP, or if their condition has symptoms that require accommodations without need for individualized education. Tics often fall in this area, and your child may need accommodations to get through the school day while managing them.

How: Just as with an IEP plan, your best bet is to reach out to your child's school psychologist. The role of a school psychologist is to know education law and legalities, and they are often the lead or point of contact in a school assessment team. They can often provide you with further information about whether looking into a 504 plan or IEP may be an option.

My Two Cents

When your child is diagnosed with a tic disorder, it can be scary. You worry about what they will do at school, how they will manage their tics, and who will be able to help them if they need it.

What if your child does not have academic difficulties, but they have challenges with emotional regulation, social skills, impulse control, or organization? Many families report to me that they are often told their child does not qualify for an IEP because they are doing fine academically. Unfortunately, school staff can often overlook and do not assess "affective needs." These needs relate to a child's social, emotional, and behavioral abilities and skills and can be associated with several of the disability categories. As we know that Tourette Syndrome falls under the umbrella of neurodiversity, it is not uncommon for children and teens with Tourette Syndrome to be considered "twice exceptional", meaning that they excel beyond the level of their peers in some areas of development while significantly falling behind them in others. Due to the nature of Tourette Syndrome, symptoms may not always be visibly apparent, and educational staff may not realize the need for support.

Federal law (IDEA) states that a free appropriate public education must be provided to all students, and those who have a health impairment (such as Tourette Syndrome) may be eligible for an IEP if the condition "adversely affects a child's educational performance."

Although school teams sometimes believe that educational performance is limited to academics, it is not. The team must also examine how the condition impacts a child's nonacademic performance. If your child is struggling in school and you are requesting an evaluation, make sure the team understands and acknowledges the following difficulties related to Tourette Syndrome, a neurological condition:

- → Disinhibition or reduced impulse control
- → Anxiety
- → Instances of rage or emotional dysregulation
- → Sensory processing differences and issues
- → Challenges with attention and focus
- → Social communication delays or deficits
- → Variable performance across environments and from day to day
- → Executive functioning delays and challenges
- → Reduced emotional maturity compared with same-age peers

If you are going through the process of an evaluation for special education or a 504 plan, you may find the following helpful:

1. Contact your local chapter of the Tourette Association. Many chapters have an education liaison who can provide information and resources to school teams and can explain some of the nuances of Tourette Syndrome that often go unrecognized in the school environment.
2. Provide the following resources to the school team:

a. https://tourette.org/resource/understanding-behavioral-symptoms-tourette-syndrome/

b. https://tourette.org/resource/iep-eligibility-is-not-only-based-on-academics/

Finally, a key skill that we often overlook in this process is the role of self-advocacy and how vital it can be in your child's school success. How will your child know when to ask to step out of the room for a tic break (even if it is on their IEP) if you don't practice that skill? How will they know how to talk about their tics with classmates who ask, "Why are you doing that?" How will they be able to manage in the classroom if they become distracted (perhaps by suppressing tics) and didn't hear the instructions for the assignment?

Before you begin the process of looking into a 504 plan or an IEP, I suggest that you take a good look at your child's ability to advocate in the school setting. For some children, once they have understood these skills (and practiced them), they are able to be successful without an IEP or 504 plan. And, to be transparent, even when students have these plans in place, teachers forget to implement the agreed upon accommodations and modifications. Or your child may have modifications in their plan, but never ask to use them. With the teenagers I work with, many of them are afraid of "looking different," and so even with a robust plan in place, they dislike using their accommodations. I completely understand.

This is a great time to have your child or teen work with an occupational therapist if you believe they need help with learning necessary assertiveness and self-advocacy skills. Even if your child's occupational therapist has no experience with tic disorders, they can help your child learn to advocate and prepare for possible roadblocks to success at school.

Here is a list of some skills that may be helpful for your child to be able to do at school, depending on age:

1. Ask for help from a teacher when they don't understand the directions or need more clarification.
2. Circle a problem they are stuck on to be able to continue to work on an activity (say on a math test). Then ask for help with the problems they need support with.
3. Plan and rehearse what to say to peers when they ask about tics in a way that feels natural to your child.
4. Know when to ask for a break to leave the room due to tics and where to go that is safe to tic. Pair this with learning how to use a watch to time the break so that it remains a helpful tool and does not transition into escape from the classroom.

If your child would be unable to do these things independently, or would need a great deal of support, that may be a clue that looking into the process for an IEP or a 504 plan is an essential next step.

As the decision to pursue the process to obtain a 504 or an IEP can be challenging, the Tourette Association of America has many free webinars and resources available on this topic. I highly suggest that, if you are considering this for your child or teen, you visit their site and spend some time reviewing some of the many valuable resources. Also, if you have a state chapter of the Tourette Association, they may have a local education liaison that can help you understand some of your options as well as provide educational resources to your child's school team.

What if you are completely overwhelmed by this process and need more individualized support? I love helping families navigate this process, and it is part of the offerings I provide in my business. What's more, I also attend 504 or IEP meetings with the family along the way so they feel comfortable with a knowledgeable expert by their side. You can find out more about these services on my website.

Workplace Accommodations for Adults

What about challenges for those in the workplace? I often receive phone calls and emails from adults related to issues at work. Some of the most challenging tics that impact a person's engagement in work or promote discrimination can include coprolalia (swearing tics) and other motor and vocal tics that appear violent or are socially inappropriate.

Research looking into quality of life overall for adults with Tourette Syndrome indicates that the combination of co-occurring conditions such as anxiety, depression, OCD, and ADHD can be difficult to manage and contribute to challenges in the workplace, especially for adults with more severe symptoms.[38] Does that mean that adults with Tourette Syndrome are doomed to a life of unemployment or underemployment? Absolutely not!

Before we dive into your legal rights in the workforce, let's first talk about how to thrive with a tic disorder as an adult.

We already know that one common challenge faced by everyone in the Tourette Syndrome community is a general lack of information by the public and the common stereotypes that abound. What can we do to combat the negative effects? A powerful tool and ally that exists is the connection to others who "get you" and can offer support and connection. You already guessed that I am going to refer you to the online (and in-person) adult support groups run by the Tourette Association of America. Did you know that they also have a group for LGBT+ individuals? For those in the UK, Tourettes Action Online also offers online groups for adults, and there is also a Tourette Syndrome Association of Australia that offers groups as well. At this time I am not aware of any other organizations worldwide that offer adult support groups, however, if you learn about any of them, please pass the info my way! If you are struggling with symptoms of your tic disorder and feel disconnected, alone, and like no one understands your journey, I recommend that you look into these groups to see if they would be a good fit for you.

For many people, the challenges that most impact them on a day-to-day basis are actually not related to tics at all but to their co-occurring conditions. If you have a diagnosis of ADHD in addition to Tourette Syndrome, you may feel that distractibility, poor focus, and disorganization are making it hard to be successful at work. Even though many of the resources available on ADHD are tailored for children, there are plenty of ways to manage your ADHD as an adult. A workbook that has been recommended to me by my clients is the book *Thriving with Adult ADHD: Skills to Strengthen Executive Functioning* by Phil Bossier. You can explore the resources and strategies in this book and implement what is helpful to you. If you are overwhelmed with where to start to manage your ADHD, there are ADHD coaches available that work with adults. These coaches can provide an evaluation of your executive functioning needs, as well as your relationship and workplace challenges. Sometimes, coaching can be a short-term endeavor, and you can always set the pace and number of sessions you feel you can commit to.

What if OCD is the concern? Finding a therapist that you relate to and feel will be a good fit can be essential. I do recommend looking for a therapist who is trained in ERP therapy—the gold standard intervention for OCD. Many clients I know also have had therapy through a website called NOCD.com, although the reviews of online therapy for OCD can be mixed, and you may prefer to find an in-person therapist.

Rights in the Workplace

Work is stressful and busy enough without also having the extra burden of figuring out and navigating your rights as someone with a tic disorder or Tourette Syndrome. Whether you are curious about your rights or experiencing difficulty in the workplace, understanding your rights is the first step.

Tourette Syndrome is a disability covered by the Americans with Disabilities Act, according to the Federal Department of Justice. Do all people with Tourette Syndrome need to assert their rights under the law? No, but if you do, this guide can walk you through the basics you need to know. In the workplace, adults with Tourette Syndrome are entitled to certain rights and protections to ensure equal opportunities and a supportive work environment.

The first thing you'll need to know is that just having a diagnosis of Tourette Syndrome or another medical condition does *not* automatically qualify you for workplace protections. You'll need to demonstrate that your symptoms are substantially limiting at least one major life activity.

While I will provide general information, it's important to note that employment laws and regulations may vary depending on your state and that this information is related to laws in the United States only. It's advisable to consult with local laws and seek legal advice specific to your situation. However, here are some general rights that you can expect based upon ADA guidelines:

Disability discrimination: Adults with Tourette Syndrome are protected under disability discrimination laws in many countries. The regulations referred to here relate to the ADA. These laws prohibit employers from discriminating against employees or job applicants based on their disability, including Tourette Syndrome. This protection extends to recruitment, hiring, promotions, job assignments, and other employment practices.

Reasonable accommodations: Employers are generally required to provide reasonable accommodations to employees with disabilities, including those with Tourette Syndrome. Reasonable accommodations are adjustments or modifications made in the workplace that allow individuals to perform their job duties effectively. Accommodations for Tourette Syndrome may include flexible work hours, a quiet workspace, or time off for medical appointments.

Disclosure: Employees are not required to disclose their Tourette Syndrome diagnosis unless they require reasonable accommodations. It's a personal decision whether or not to disclose your condition to your employer or colleagues. However, if you need accommodations, it may be necessary to disclose your condition to request the appropriate support.

Confidentiality: Employers are generally required to keep an employee's medical information confidential. This means that information about your Tourette Syndrome should be shared only with individuals who have a legitimate need to know, such as human resources personnel or supervisors involved in providing accommodations.

Are you looking for information about a specific situation or for a specific state? Try Googling "disability law" plus your state to find local resource centers and agencies in your area.

CONCLUSION

I almost didn't write this book. It sat on my heart for years, and I kept thinking about how helpful it would be for people. I read all the other books on Amazon about managing tics, and I knew there was a need for a book written by a therapist who helps people with tics daily and with tools they could use immediately. Finally, I started writing.

I had this quote on my desk, and read it every day when I worked on this book:

> "If one person can learn from the things you experienced that can change their life, that is worth documenting the process."
>
> —RUSSELL BRUNSON

This quote inspired me to keep going, wanting to offer actionable tools that people could use today to begin flourishing with tics, to begin regaining their lives and confidence.

Now it is your turn. Take what you have learned in this book, and try something new to implement. And write to me and tell me about it! I really want to hear about your successes. If you recognize that you want (or need) more support than a book can offer, I welcome you to contact me via email (mary@helpfortics.com) or look at the services on my website that are specifically tailored for people with tic disorders. My promise to you is that I will help you manage your tics in the most effective and efficient way possible. If you are ready to start your own journey, you can reach me at my website here: www.helpfortics.com.

If you only take away one thing from this book, understand that you are unique, even if your diagnosis is not. Just as no one in the world has the same fingerprints as you do, your neurological signatures and neural connections are distinctive to you. We have not yet discovered all of the magic of the human brain; in fact, we have just scratched the surface. Insights and discoveries related to the concept of neuroplasticity (the ability of the brain to change) are expanding daily. It is my greatest wish that you will know how special you are and that you are not "broken," just extraordinary. Never give up on your own journey for the best life for you, no matter what *anyone* says.

ACKNOWLEDGEMENTS

This book would not be possible without the inspiration from my clients. If we have ever worked together, or if I have ever had the honor of supporting your child, you encouraged me to write this book. Thank you from the bottom of my heart.

Jeremy and Jacki, thank you both for reminding me that I had enough to say to make a difference.

To the Arizona Chapter of the Tourette Association, Kris, Deanna, and Hillary, thank you for welcoming me into your fold and for your dedication to ensuring people with tic disorders have support and connection.

To Dr. Poonam Bhatia and Dr. David Shprecher, you are rare among neurologists in your compassion, enthusiasm, and expertise for the community you serve. The people of Arizona are so fortunate to have you. Grateful for your endless work and the wisdom you impart.

APPENDIX A: OTHER OPTIONS FOR TIC MANAGEMENT

As soon as your child started having tics, you likely headed directly to Google. One of the first treatments to pop up in your search engine to stop tics was probably this evidence-based therapy, Comprehensive Behavioral Intervention for Tics, or CBIT for short. CBIT is recommended by the American Academy of Neurology as a first-line therapy for people with tics and can be used whether or not you or your child is taking medication. But should everyone try CBIT therapy, and what is it really like? Let's answer those questions, and no, this is not a sales pitch but my honest professional opinion about CBIT.

What is CBIT?

CBIT is a therapy for tics that originated from a type of behavioral therapy called Habit Reversal Therapy. This therapy has five core components: awareness training (bringing attention to the sensations and behaviors), function-based intervention (determine what makes the tics more likely and what could be reinforcing them), competing response training (creating a different behavior or movement to alter the tic cycle), relaxation training (learning skills to calm the body and mind), and generalization training (learning to apply the skills in all situations).

It usually is recommended for six to eight weeks consecutively then tapered off depending on the progress of the person.

Is CBIT only for children?

No. Adults of all ages, teens, and children can benefit, even if they have had tics for years. The oldest client I have guided through CBIT was in her late fifties, and the youngest client I've had was a mature seven-year-old. Standard CBIT is often not recommended for children under seven or eight years of age, although other therapy options may help, such as counseling or occupational therapy.

What can I expect from CBIT?

Here is where we need to be realistic and share the honest, true expectations about what you may get from CBIT therapy. The best possible outcome is that tics go away completely or are significantly reduced. In my years of helping people with CBIT, I have only had a few clients that was the case for. For most clients, you can expect that your tics will be more manageable (in many cases significantly). You can be 100 percent sure that you will learn more about your hidden personal tic triggers, how the tic cycle works, and how to modify things in your life to make them less severe. You will definitely learn calming and coping strategies that you can rely on when your tics flare, and that benefit alone can improve your quality of life.

Should everyone do CBIT?

Simply put, no. If you are currently experiencing significant anxiety, OCD, or depression, you are likely not a good candidate. If you have ADHD that makes it very difficult for you to focus and impossible to control impulses, you are likely not a good candidate. Why not? The reason is because, as CBIT is a behavioral therapy, it requires participation and follow-through on the part of the participant. It requires tracking tics (with help) and growing a window of tolerance for discomfort and change. I always tell parents that I want to be as sure as I can that a child will be successful. I'd much rather delay the start of a rigorous CBIT program than take on a client who is not ready. I don't want to waste a person's time (or money), or worse, have a person feel that they have "failed" if they didn't have much success.

Another reason CBIT may not be right for you at this time is if you are going through a big life change (divorce, change in family structure, stressful new job). These changes can cause your stress level to increase (obviously!) and make tics much harder to manage.

What is the evidence behind CBIT?

Are you wondering if there is any evidence to back up the claims of the effectiveness of Comprehensive Behavioral Intervention for Tics? As we've already stated, not every person will respond to CBIT in the same way, but the studies completed back up the American Academy of Neurology's recommendation that it should be a first-line treatment. A 2010 randomized controlled trial published in the *Journal of the American Medical Association* found that children receiving CBIT therapy compared with the control group (who received supportive psychotherapy and education only) significantly reduced their scores on a baseline assessment of tic severity (Yale Global Tic Severity Scale) than the control group. And what's more, 87 percent of the children who responded positively to the therapy continued to benefit six months following the treatment.[39]

We've already done CBIT, and it wasn't very helpful. Why not?

As I've stated before, it is important to make sure that a person is really ready for CBIT. They also must want to participate for it to be effective. If a parent is requesting CBIT, but their child is not aware of their tics or does not want to try it, it is not recommended to to proceed with therapy at that time.

Another reason your therapy may have not been helpful is because you needed another type of treatment. For some people, their tics are at a level of severity that CBIT is not enough. If you are not sure if CBIT is for you, it's a good idea to discuss the next best steps with a CBIT therapist and your neurologist.

Finally, not all CBIT therapists are the same. People with varied professional backgrounds can be providers of CBIT, and each provider has a different level of expertise. No matter what type of therapy you pursue, you should always ask questions about your therapist's background, expertise, and outcomes.

How do I find a CBIT provider?

If you live in the vicinity of a Tourette Center of Excellence, the providers there can often refer you to a CBIT therapist and may even have some on staff. What if you don't live near one? One way to go about finding a provider is to go to the Tourette.org website and search for provider listings. If you are a member of several of the available Facebook groups focusing on tics and tic disorders, you may also ask for a recommendation from a family or individual that has used a specific provider.

Find an Occupational Therapist Who Is Experienced in the Areas You Need

Another step I recommend to my clients and to people in the Tourette Syndrome and tic community for tic management is to find an occupational therapist. Speaking of occupational therapy, if you don't know what occupational therapy is (and that's okay, most people don't) and why occupational therapists can help people with tic disorders, let me tell you about my profession and what we offer.

Occupational therapists are health professionals who help a person get back to (or develop the skills for) participation in essential life activities (called "occupations"). This can be as broad as being able to dress, eat, and shower post stroke or injury, problem solving executive functioning delays in a child with ADHD who is struggling in school with turning in homework, to addressing sensory challenges with an autistic child. We often work in school settings, therapy clinics, and hospitals.

Because we have such a large scope, it is imperative that you find an occupational therapist who can help you with the specific barriers that you need to overcome. Not all occupational therapists are the same and have the same level of experience. Why do I recommend starting with an occupational therapist after diagnosis? Here are some of the ways that an occupational therapist can help you if you have a tic disorder:

1. **Emotional regulation:** Occupational therapists are experts in helping individuals and families learn new methods and techniques for emotional regulation. As we've seen in the Tourette Syndrome iceberg, challenges with bursts of rage, impulsivity, and reduced emotional regulation are common. Find someone who has experience in this area if this is one of the barriers to success for your family.

2. **Setting up routines that work:** Often, especially in families, the day-to-day routines and responsibilities are not efficient and can contribute to stress. Sometimes, parents have resorted to doing tasks for their children in order to simplify things and just get out the door on time. If this is you, don't worry! This is a common way for parents to cope, and we know you do the best you can with what you've got. An occupational therapist can analyze and observe the current state of your household and can coach you in making needed changes.

3. **Addressing sensory processing needs:** Whether you (or your child) is demonstrating some sensory hypersensitivity or are wondering if sensory inputs are playing a role in triggering your tics, this is our jam! As we learned, at minimum screening for the ways in which sensory inputs and modulation are affecting tics and function is essential for a successful tic management plan. Why not go to the best professionals in this area?

4. **Poor sleep:** Whether your sleep is compromised due to tics, poor sleep patterns, or sensory dysregulation, learning ways

to improve your sleep is essential for basic well-being. And, as you can imagine, lack of quality sleep impacts your ability to manage tics. Evidence shows that people with Tourette Syndrome demonstrate more difficulty with sleep in general, as well as have persistent limb movements during sleep.[40] There is also a great deal of research about sleep dysfunction and its correlation with ADHD (24). An occupational therapist can help with the creation of new sleep routines as well as techniques for movement-based challenges in sleep, such as restless legs.

5. **Managing executive function delays and lagging skills:** Another area occupational therapists can specialize in is the treatment of ADHD and often connected lagging executive functioning skills. This realm is typically thought of as being related to children, but I will tell you that I have an increasing number of adults who are wanting to address their chronic disorganization, lateness, and task overwhelm. If you are not familiar with what executive functioning skills are, the term comes from the idea that the frontal cortex of our brain is the executive function of the brain and therefore has to manage the essential "boss jobs." These "jobs" include memory, planning, self-control, problem solving, cognitive flexibility, attention, time management, emotional regulation, and inhibitory control. Sound like any areas you or your child is struggling with? Find an occupational therapist near you who specializes in this—STAT!

I hope these examples have helped you see why I always recommend having an occupational therapist as part of your treatment team. Looking for an occupational therapist is one of the first steps I'd start with after diagnosis. But how do you choose one? They all seem the same. You don't want to waste time with a provider who can't help. Let me give you some questions to ask when you interview an occupational therapist.

Questions to Ask an Occupational Therapist

1. Do you have any experience with Tourette Syndrome or tic disorders? (They likely won't; there are not many with expertise in this area. But they don't need to be for your purposes. You are looking for someone to address the barriers to other occupations first.)

2. Do you involve your clients in setting their own goals and determining the direction of their therapy (if appropriate)?

3. Do you (and will you) collaborate with other professionals, such as speech therapists, psychologists, or neurologists, when working with clients?

4. Do you have any specialties? I am looking for someone with expertise in (ADHD, learning disabilities, executive functioning disorders, your specific needs). No need to be fancy, just use plain English and describe the outcomes you'd like to see.

5. How do you promote progress in the home environment after the session is over? What are some typical homework or home programs that you recommend?

6. What is your expertise in the area of sensory processing? Can you describe your approach?

7. What are some of the programs, curriculum, and frameworks that you use for emotional regulation? How effective are they?

8. How do you measure progress and know where to take your interventions? Do you involve your clients in this process?

9. What will our communication be like during therapy, and how frequently do you recommend we communicate?

10. How do you involve family members or caregivers in the therapy process??

APPENDIX B: UNDERSTANDING FUNCTIONAL TICS AND FUNCTIONAL NEUROLOGICAL DISORDER

Since the COVID-19 pandemic, there has been a massive increase in awareness and diagnosis of a condition called Functional Neurological Disorder (FND).[41] One of the initial symptoms is sometimes tics, although they are different from the tics you have with a diagnosis of Tourette Syndrome. The symptoms of FND can impact the motor system, the sensory system, areas of cognition, and psychological well-being.

One of the most challenging aspects of FND is actually getting the diagnosis. Unfortunately, because there are so many symptoms that seem to be disparate at first glance, it often takes a long time (and many ER visits and specialists) for a person to actually get the diagnosis of FND. And here's the kicker, when you do actually get the diagnosis, most doctors don't have any treatment options for you. In the past, there has even been disagreement within the medical community about whether psychiatry or neurology is the right discipline to treat this disorder. This means that people with FND often get shuffled between specialists, with little clarity and actionable treatment steps.

What are the symptoms of Functional Neurological Disorder, how do they differ from the symptoms of Tourette Syndrome?[42] [43] Let's compare and contrast them with a table:

Functional Neurological Disorder	Tourette Syndrome
→ Presence of tics	→ Presence of tics
→ Anxiety often co-occurring	→ Anxiety often co-occurring
→ ADHD not often co-occurring	→ ADHD often co-occurring
→ OCD not often co-occurring	→ OCD often co-occurring
→ Tics are often highly variable	→ Tics are often stereotyped
→ Tics often complex	→ Tics can be simple or complex
→ Age at onset older (late childhood or teen years)	→ Usual age at onset early childhood
→ More likely to be female	→ More likely to be male
→ Less likely to have premonitory urge	→ More likely to have premonitory urge
→ Symptoms tend to respond to intentional distractibility	→ Symptoms do not tend to respond to intentional distractibility
→ Typically no family history of tics	→ Often a family history of tics
→ Tics begin suddenly with great severity	→ Generally begins gradually with mild facial tics
→ Often history of trauma	→ History of trauma not likely
→ More likely to experience self-injurious tics	→ Less likely to experience self-injurious tics
→ More likely to experience tics with socially unacceptable words or gestures	→ Less likely to experience tics with socially unacceptable words or gestures
→ More likely to have tics that impact voluntary actions (blocking or freezing tics)	→ Less likely to have tics that impact voluntary actions (blocking tics)

As you can see from the table, there are quite a few differences between so-called "functional tics" and "organic tics." But no matter what you call them, is there anything you can do about them? Many people have heard of CBIT therapy, and it is recommended as a first-line treatment for tics. But what about functional tics? What can we do about them?

At this time, there is sparse information outlining a specific and robust treatment approach to FND as well as functional tics. The good news is that new research is coming out daily as the number of people with these diagnoses rises. Research has indicated that the best way to help a person with FND reduce their symptoms is by using a multidisciplinary approach, with incorporation of physical therapy for movement and motor symptoms, psychology and psychiatry for emotional regulation, and occupational therapy for problem solving barriers to life, cognitive challenges, regulating the autonomic nervous system, as well as addressing changes in sensory processing. [44] [45]

Based on the symptoms of FND, the following are the topics I ask a person or family about after they have a diagnosis of FND and come to me for therapy:

1. **Sensory symptoms:** Do you have any sensory differences or changes in tolerance that have made things difficult for you? (Ex: greater sensitivity to sound or light, reactions to smells are different, etc.)

2. **Tic symptoms:** Do you have any tics that are bothering you? Which ones are bothering you the most? Are any of them painful?

3. **Emotional processing symptoms:** What is your self-regulation and mood like? Has anything changed in the way you cope with stressors or how you engage in new situations?

4. **Activity/occupation symptoms:** Are you able to do the things you used to do? How successful are you with basic things, like self-care, meal preparation, and cleaning up after yourself, right now? What about more complex things, such as going to new places, driving a car, or shopping for groceries?

5. **Cognitive symptoms:** How are you doing in school or work? When you need to learn new things or read, what is your comprehension like? Are you forgetting things often? Do you experience brain fog?

Most of these symptoms can be addressed by an occupational therapist with knowledge and experience in working with functional disorders. But what about the tics? Many of my clients have made progress with their most distressing tics using CBIT therapy (or components of it), even though there is no clear evidence of its effectiveness with functional tics at this time.

As the treatment of FND can be a book in itself, here are my brief recommendations for you if you have been diagnosed with FND:

1. Put together the members of your multidisciplinary team. This includes psychiatry and psychology, physical therapy, occupational therapy, and neurology. It is best if you grant permission for all team members to communicate so that they can work together, or at least update each other on your progress. If you have a team member that will not agree to this, find a new one!

2. If you are experiencing functional tics, find a CBIT therapist, and let them know of your diagnosis so that they can adapt the strategies as needed.

3. Examine with your therapist whether you need school or work accommodations. Have them recommend some possible accommodations based upon your symptoms. (Caveat here: ensure that symptoms will not be inadvertently reinforced and are only used as necessary.)

APPENDIX C: FREQUENTLY ASKED QUESTIONS

Now that you have read this book, you may have a list of questions that have come to mind—ones that you want answers to, now! I want to provide you with evidence-based answers to common questions that my clients have, along with my clinical opinions and experiences as a provider who works with people with tic disorders daily.

My doctor says we should just "wait and see." I don't want to do that. What can we do today?

When you are going to a primary care doctor, pediatrician, or neurologist for the first time, and your child's tics started within the last few months, you may be told to adopt a "wait and see" approach. The reason for this is because some tics can be transient, with up to 20 percent of young children having temporary tics during childhood. This can be frustrating and distressing for both parents and children, who were hoping to receive some definitive information and concrete next steps. It can be enough to leave you lying awake in bed or continually Googling what to do. But guess what! There are things you can do, starting today.

You can try CBIT. As we discussed previously, CBIT is recommended as a first-line therapy by the AAN. It can be used with children and adults and can be effective with tic disorders of many types, including temporary or transient tics. You can use the strategies and tools in this book. Finally, you can join your area's chapter of the Tourette Association to connect with other families who understand what you are going through and can provide support.

How can outside factors influence tics? Aren't they involuntary?

This is a question that my clients' families often ask me at our first sessions. And it is a great one! There is emerging evidence that both sympathetic and parasympathetic nervous activity influences tic expression. You may know these parts of our autonomic nervous system as the "fight or flight" or "rest and digest" system. In plain English, this means that anything that excites or increases arousal of our sympathetic nervous system has the potential to trigger tics, whether it is stressful or fun and exciting. Some of the pharmacological treatments which act on sympathetic tone are often helpful. For example, clonidine is often used as a first-choice medication for treating TS in children. Clonidine suppresses sympathetic activity and can reduce the triggering of motor tics. Beyond medication, you can influence the function of the sympathetic nervous system with simple strategies discussed in the sensory sections previously.

How do we cope with tics in public?

Having loud vocal and visible motor tics in public can be distressing and sometimes embarrassing. It can be annoying when people stare and can make a person with tics limit their activities. Don't let this happen to you. The Tourette Association of America has an excellent resource about how to manage tics in public. Here are their recommendations:

→ Carry an "I have Tourette Syndrome" card or wear a medical ID bracelet.
→ Don't isolate yourself.
→ Bring something attention absorbing; take advantage of that attentional flashlight strategy!
→ Bring a friend.
→ Be prepared.
→ Prepare others.
→ Frame your response.
→ Seek opportunities.

Can you have both Functional Neurological Disorder and Tourette Syndrome at the same time?

Yes, you can. Having a diagnosis of both FND and TS is less common, but it does happen. It can be tricky, as having both disorders may make you feel like you "don't belong" anywhere. There are support groups for all ages with Tourette Syndrome, but accessing groups for people with FND is much harder. Please know that if you have a dual diagnosis, it doesn't make your experiences with tics any less "real" or "valid." Most in the medical field are moving away from the Conversion Disorder terminology, as it can lead people to believe that their symptoms are related to emotionality. There is also the possibility that a person diagnosed with it may feel a sense of self-blame due to the way it is often explained to the patient. Professionals are starting to recognize this to ensure that people diagnosed with FND understand that, although there may be a psychological basis for some people, it is not a required component for the diagnosis. There are measurable neurological signs and markers that correspond with the diagnosis, and recent research related to brain imaging indicates changes in functional connectivity within specific areas of the brain.[46]

Is Comprehensive Behavioral Therapy for Tics a neurodiversity-affirming therapy?

Absolutely! Many of the clients I see have multiple diagnoses, and the number of people with both ASD and TS is increasing. As we noted before, current CDC data reports that, as of 2020, approximately one in thirty-six children has a diagnosis of autism.[47] And, no, it is not simply because we are getting better at diagnosing. For people that have any type of neurodevelopmental disorder (including ADHD and learning disorders), it is imperative to ensure that we are approaching therapy from a neurodiversity-affirming mindset. If you are not familiar with the term, it simply means that therapy should validate the unique way a person connects with and experiences the world based on their individual neurological makeup.

CBIT therapy, although it allows us to target tics and things we would like to change or improve, encourages a person to examine how their tics impact them directly and whether (or not) they want to address a particular tic. During the course of therapy, we help the person decide what is important to them, and self-advocacy surrounding their needs is part of the process!

ENDNOTES

1   Centers for Disease Control and Prevention. (May 4, 2023). Tourette Syndrome Data and Statistics. https://www.cdc.gov/ncbddd/tourette/data.html.

2   American Academy of Neurology. (May 6, 2019). New AAN Guideline for Treating Tourette Syndrome and Other Chronic Disorders. Press release. https://www.aan.com/PressRoom/Home/PressRelease/2721.

3   Shprecher, D. R., Rubenstein, L. A., Gannon, K., Frank, S. A., & Kurlan, R. (2014). Temporal course of the Tourette syndrome clinical triad. Tremor and Other Hyperkinetic Movements, 4, 243. https://doi.org/10.7916/D8HD7SV6.

4   Zimmerman, M. (1986). Neurophysiology of Sensory Systems. In R. F. Schmidt (Ed.), Fundamentals of Sensory Physiology (pp. 68-116). Springer. https://doi.org/10.1007/978-3-642-82598-9_3.

5   Ranford, J., MacLean, J., Alluri, P. R., Comeau, O., Godena, E., LaFrance Jr, W. C., Hunt, A., Stephen, C. D., & Perez, D. L. (2020). Sensory Processing Difficulties in Functional Neurological Disorder: A Possible Predisposing Vulnerability? Psychosomatics, 61(4), 343–352. https://doi.org/10.1016/j.psym.2020.02.003.

6   Houghton, D. C., Capriotti, M. R., Conelea, C. A., & Woods, D. W. (2014). Sensory Phenomena in Tourette Syndrome: Their Role in Symptom Formation and Treatment. *Current Developmental Disorders Reports*, 1(4), 245–251. https://doi.org/10.1007/s40474-014-0026-2.

7   Scahill, L., Lombroso, P. J., Mack, G., Van Wattum, P. J., Zhang, H., Vitale, A., & Leckman, J. F. (2001). Thermal Sensitivity in Tourette syndrome: Preliminary Report. *Perceptual and Motor Skills*, 92(2), 419-432. https://doi.org/10.2466/pms.2001.92.2.419.

8   Belluscio, B. A., Jin, L., Watters, V., Lee, T. H., & Hallett, M. (2011). Sensory sensitivity to external stimuli in Tourette syndrome patients. *Movement Disorders*, 26(14), 2538–2543. https://doi.org/10.1002/mds.23977.

9   Woods, D. W., Watson, T. S., Wolfe, E., Twohig, M. P., & Friman, P. C. (2001). Analyzing the influence of tic-related talk on vocal and motor tics in children with Tourette's syndrome. *Journal of Applied Behavior Analysis*, 34(3), 353-356. doi:10.1901/jaba.2001.34-353.

10   van Dijk, J. G., Koenderink, M., Kramer, C. G. S., den Heijer, J. C., & Roos, R. A. C. (1992). Non-invasive assessment of autonomic nervous function in Gilles de la Tourette syndrome. *Clinical Neurology and Neurosurgery*, 94(2), 157-159. https://doi.org/10.1016/0303-8467(92)90074-D.

11   Leisman, G., & Sheldon, D. (2022). Tics and Emotions. *Brain Sciences*, 12(2), 242. https://doi.org/10.3390/brainsci12020242.

12   Nagai, Y., Cavanna, A., & Critchley, H. D. (2009). Influence of sympathetic autonomic arousal on tics: Implications for a therapeutic behavioral intervention for Tourette syndrome. *Journal of Psychosomatic Research*, 67, 599–605.

13   Rădulescu, A., Herron, J., Kennedy, C., et al. (2017). Global and local excitation and inhibition shape the dynamics of the cortico-striatal-thalamo-cortical pathway. *Scientific Reports*, 7, 7608.

14   Buckner, R. L., Andrews-Hanna, J. R., & Schacter, D. L. (2008). The brain's default network - anatomy, function, and relevance to disease. *Annals of the New York Academy of Sciences*, 1124, 1–38.

15   Seeley, W. W. (2019). The salience network: A neural system for perceiving and responding to homeostatic demands. *Journal of Neuroscience*, 39(50), 9878–9882.

16   Sigurdsson, H. P., Jackson, S. R., Jolley, L., Mitchell, E., & Jackson, G. M. (2020). Alterations in cerebellar grey matter structure and covariance networks in young people with Tourette syndrome. *Cortex*, 126, 1-15.

17   Doja, A., Bookwala, A., Pohl, D., Rossi-Ricci, A., Barrowman, N., Chan, J., & Longmuir, P. E. (2018). Relationship Between Physical Activity, Tic Severity and Quality of Life in Children with Tourette Syndrome. *Journal of the Canadian Academy of Child and Adolescent Psychiatry*, 27(4), 222–227.

18   Kim, D., Warburton, D., Wu, N., Barr, A., Honer, W., & Procyshyn, R. (2018). Effects of physical activity on the symptoms of Tourette syndrome: A systematic review. *European Psychiatry*, 48(1), 13-19.

19   Anderson, E., & Shivakumar, G. (2013). Effects of exercise and physical activity on anxiety. *Frontiers in Psychiatry*, 4, 27.

20   Bowman, K. (2014). Move Your DNA: Restore Your Health Through Natural Movement. Victory Belt Publishing.

21   Miguel, E. C., do Rosário-Campos, M. C., Prado, H. S., do Valle, R., Rauch, S. L., Coffey, B. J., Baer, L., Savage, C. R., O'Sullivan, R. L., Jenike, M. A., & Leckman, J. F. (2000). Sensory phenomena in obsessive-compulsive disorder and Tourette's disorder. *Journal of Clinical Psychiatry*, 61(2), 150-156.

22   Patel, N., Jankovic, J., & Hallett, M. (2014). Sensory aspects of movement disorders. *The Lancet Neurology*, 13(1), 100–112.

23   Biermann-Ruben, K., Miller, A., Franzkowiak, S., et al. (2012). Increased sensory feedback in Tourette syndrome. *NeuroImage*, 63(1), 119–125.

24   Eley, T. C., Stirling, L., Ehlers, A., Gregory, A. M., & Clark, D. M. (2004). Heart-beat perception, panic/somatic symptoms and anxiety sensitivity in children. *Behaviour Research and Therapy*, 42(4), 439-448.

25   Sleep Foundation. (n.d.). Noise and Sleep. Retrieved from https://www.sleepfoundation.org/noise-and-sleep/white-noise.

26   Kawada, T., & Suzuki, S. (1993). Sleep induction effects of steady 60 dB (A) pink noise. *Industrial Health*, 31, 35–38.

27   Hardian, H., Febriani, S. S., Sumekar, T. A., Muniroh, M., Indraswari, D. A., Purwoko, Y., & Ambarwati, E. (2020). Improvement of Sleep Quality by Autonomous Sensory Meridian Response (ASMR) Stimulation Among Medical Students. *Malaysian Journal of Medical and Health Sciences*, 16, 81–85.

28   Lee, M., Lee, H. J., Ahn, J., Hong, J. K., & Yoon, I. Y. (2022). Comparison of autonomous sensory meridian response and binaural

auditory beats effects on stress reduction: a pilot study. *Scientific Reports*, 12(1), 19521.

29 Kawai, H., Kishimoto, M., Okahisa, Y., Sakamoto, S., Terada, S., & Takaki, M. (2023). Initial Outcomes of the Safe and Sound Protocol on patients with adult autism spectrum disorder: Exploratory Pilot Study. *International Journal of Environmental Research and Public Health*, 20(6), 4862.

30 Ricketts, E. J., Burgess, H. J., Montalbano, G. E., Coles, M. E., McGuire, J. F., Thamrin, H., McMakin, D. L., McCracken, J. T., Carskadon, M. A., Piacentini, J., & Colwell, C. S. (2022). Morning light therapy in adults with Tourette's disorder. *Journal of Neurology*, 269(1), 399–410.

31 Retimer. (n.d.). https://www.re-timer.com.

32 Afif, I. Y., Manik, A. R., Munthe, K., et al. (2022). Physiological Effect of Deep Pressure in Reducing Anxiety of Children with ASD during Traveling: A Public Transportation Setting. *Bioengineering* (Basel, Switzerland), 9(4), 157.

33 Meth, E. M. S., Brandão, L. E. M., van Egmond, L. T., et al. (2023). A weighted blanket increases pre-sleep salivary concentrations of melatonin in young, healthy adults. *Journal of Sleep Research*, 32(2), e13743.

34 Gobbel, R. (2023). *Raising Kids with Big, Baffling Behaviors*. Jessica Kingsley Publishers.

35 Kaido, T., Hirabayashi, H., Murase, N., Sasaki, R., Shimokawara, T., Nagata, K., Bando, C., & Aono, Y. (2020). Deep slow nasal respiration

with tight lip closure for immediate attenuation of severe tics. *Journal of Clinical Neuroscience*, 77, 67-74.

36   Russo, MA, Santarelli DM, O'Rourke D. The physiological effects of slow breathing in the healthy human. *Breathe*, 13: 298-309.

37   Włodarczyk, A., Cubała, W. J., & Wielewicka, A. (2020). Ketogenic Diet: A Dietary Modification as an Anxiolytic Approach? *Nutrients*, 12(12), 3822.

38   Eapen, V., Cavanna, A. E., & Robertson, M. M. (2016). Comorbidities, Social Impact, and Quality of Life in Tourette Syndrome. *Frontiers in Psychiatry*, 7, 97.

39   Piacentini, J., Woods, D. W., Scahill, L., et al. (2010). Behavior Therapy for Children With Tourette Disorder: A Randomized Controlled Trial. *JAMA*, 303(19), 1929–1937. doi:10.1001/jama.2010.607.

40   Jiménez-Jiménez, F. J., Alonso-Navarro, H., García-Martín, E., & Agúndez, J. A. G. (2022). Sleep Disorders and Sleep Problems in Patients With Tourette Syndrome and Other Tic Disorders: Current Perspectives. *Nature and Science of Sleep*, 14, 1313–1331.

41   Pringsheim, T., Ganos, C., McGuire, J. F., Hedderly, T., Woods, D., Gilbert, D. L., Piacentini, J., Dale, R. C., Martino, D. (2021). Rapid Onset Functional Tic-Like Behaviors in Young Females During the COVID-19 Pandemic. *Movement Disorders*, 36(12), 2707-2713.

42   Andersen, K., Jensen, I., Okkels, K. B., Skov, L., & Debes, N. M. (2023). Clarifying the Differences between Patients with Organic Tics and Functional Tic-Like Behaviors. *Healthcare*, 11(10), 1481.

43   Ganos, C., Martino, D., Espay, A. J., Lang, A. E., Bhatia, K. P., & Edwards, M. J. (2019). Tics and functional tic-like movements: Can we tell them apart? *Neurology*, 93(17), 750-758.

44   Nicholson, C., Edwards, M. J., Carson, A. J., et al. (2020). Occupational therapy consensus recommendations for functional neurological disorder. *Journal of Neurology, Neurosurgery & Psychiatry*, 91, 1037-1045.

45   Paredes-Echeverri, S., Maggio, J., Bègue, I., Pick, S., Nicholson, T. R., & Perez, D. L. (2021). Autonomic, endocrine, and inflammation profiles in functional neurological disorder: A systematic review and meta-analysis. *Psychosomatics*, 61(4), 343–352. https://doi.org/10.1016/j.psym.2020.02.003.

46   Kozlowska, K., Spooner, C. J., Palmer, D. M., Harris, A., Korgaonkar, M. S., Scher, S., Williams, L. M. (2018). "Motoring in idle": The default mode and somatomotor networks are overactive in children and adolescents with functional neurological symptoms. *NeuroImage: Clinical*, 18, 730-743.

47   Centers for Disease Control and Prevention. (2023, March 22). Autism prevalence higher, according to data from 11 ADDM communities. Retrieved August 18, 2023. https://www.cdc.gov/media/releases/2023/p0323-autism.html.

ABOUT THE AUTHOR:

Mary Shouse, M.S. OTR/L is an occupational therapist with a passion for helping people with tic disorders live their best lives. As a provider of a therapy called Comprehensive Behavioral Intervention for Tics and a specialist in tic disorders, she has helped clients of all ages increase their confidence and reduce tics.

Mary's innovative approach combines the use of biofeedback, anxiety management, and self-awareness for progress that is medication-free. She uses a neurodiversity-affirming approach in her work and supports people to be their authentic selves in therapy and life.

Mary holds a master's in occupational therapy from A.T. Still University as well as a degree in special education from Arizona State University. A lifelong volunteer, she has served as the youth ambassador coordinator for the Arizona Chapter of the Tourette Association since 2019 as well as a past advocate for youth and teens in foster care. She adores her long-haired guinea pigs, drinking too much coffee, and shopping at Aldi.

You can visit Mary online at www.helpfortics.com or on Instagram @empowered.over.tics.

Milton Keynes UK
Ingram Content Group UK Ltd.
UKHW020740080124
435661UK00017B/1109